Psychiatry for Beginners

*Dedicated to the students
of neuroscience:
past, present & future*

Psychiatry for Beginners

Ravi Gupta MD, PhD, MAMS
Certified Sleep Physician (World Sleep Federation)
Associate Professor
Department of Psychiatry and Sleep Clinic
Himalayan Institute of Medical Sciences
Dehradun, Uttrakhand

ELSEVIER

ELSEVIER

RELX India Private Limited

Registered Office: 818, 8th Floor, Indraprakash Building, 21, Barakhamba Road, New Delhi 110001
Corporate Office: 14th Floor, Building No. 10B, DLF Cyber City, Phase II, Gurgaon-122002, Haryana, India

---

Psychiatry for Beginners, 1e, Gupta

Notice

Manager—Content Strategy: Renu Rawat
Content Strategist (Digital): Nabajyoti Kar
Manager—Education Solutions (Digital): Smruti Snigdha
Sr Project Manager—Education Solutions: Shabina Nasim
Content Development Specialist: Shravan Kumar
Project Manager: Nayagi Athmanathan
Cover Designer: Milind Majgaonkar

Typeset by GW India
Printed in India by Rajkamal Electric Press, Kundli, Haryana.

Foreword

Psychiatry is now an undergraduate teaching subject. The students joining MBBS course are taught psychiatry through lectures, seminars and clinical posting. In some institutions, the duration is up to 40 hours during the entire period. In addition, the understanding is enhanced through posting in the department of Psychiatry during internship. It is thus essential that the students have a book to refer to. It is in this context the current book is relevant.

To many, psychiatry is an esoteric subject far removed from traditional medicine and is the step-child of medicine. Dr. Jeffrey A. Lieberman, MD, past President (2000) of the American Psychiatric Association in his book "Shrinks: The Untold Story of Psychiatry, 2015" addresses the journey from rural asylum to the general hospital—Psychiatry reborn - Out of the wilderness - The brain revolution. The pendulum swing was from illness of the mind to illness of the brain. The American Psychiatric Association (APA) in 1970s stated clearly that mental illness is a medical disorder. The book went further to add that the heart is merely a glorified pump. It was proposed that brain controlled specific functions and their malfunction causes mental illness. Furthermore, the advent of CT scan (1976), MRI (1981), PET scan (1997) and fMRI pointed towards neuronal circuits and neurotransmitter. *Biological psychiatrists were born.* With the advancement of medicines (psychopharmacology), the patients were getting well.

It is imperative that the young learners are exposed to these issues and the foundation to biological basis of psychiatric illness is laid. The readers would find answers to some of these questions in this book. Hope they would enjoy and benefit!

Prof. Rajat Ray
Head, Department of Psychiatry
Himalyan Institute of Medical Sciences
Dehradun, Uttrakhand

Preface

Medicine is an ever-changing science, and we have witnessed a great progress in the diagnostic and therapeutics over past 50 years in every branch of medicine. Psychiatry is not an exception, and it has witnessed a phenomenal change in the diagnostic and therapeutic techniques over past 30 years. What was once considered as psychological is now seen as neurobiological. This has brought a phenomenal change in learning and practice of Psychiatry.

Despite advancement, our understanding of the functional aspects of the brain is still limited. Though we have initial insights to the brain areas that govern behaviour, emotions and cognition, still the existing knowledge can best be considered as patchy and far from complete. This is one reason that description of psychiatric disorders always remained descriptive or observation based. However, the latest classification system of psychiatric disorders (DSM-5) has tried to incorporate neurobiological data for the categorization and description of psychiatric disorders. This system has been followed as the backbone in this book. Thus, this book follows the neurobiological approach to the understanding of psychiatric disorders and their treatment.

Owing to the limited information regarding functional aspects of the brain, the existing neurobiological models are quite complex. At the same time, complexity also reflects the intricacies of the neurotransmitter pathways of the brain and their interaction. Considering the scope of the book, the models have been kept as simple as possible. Readers must understand that these models may change over time with the advancement of information.

This book also intends to conceptualize Psychiatry among readers and to facilitate this, basic concept of disease has been presented in the initial paragraph of every chapter. This book also compares the nosology and clinical presentation between two major classification systems (ICD-10 and DSM-5) so as to apprise you with changing concepts of classification. This will also allow you to appear in various examinations as DSM-5 is followed in USA while other countries prefer ICD-10 classification system.

The clinic-based approach has been adopted in this book rather than the textbook approach. This is why each chapter runs back from the vignette to the description of clinical features and then pathophysiology. Besides differential diagnosis, a section on diagnostic fallacies has been provided in each chapter. This has been added to make you well verse with the subject in the clinical practice. To make it further useful for the clinical practice, basic outlines of the management of disorders have also been provided.

This book is divided into various sections that are the existing sub-specialties in Psychiatry. Repetition of content has been avoided not just within the book but also through exclusion of the information accessible through other textbooks of Medical undergraduate program. This is one reason that section on Psychopharmacology primarily deals with mechanisms of action and mechanisms of adverse effects rather than pharmacological profile of psychotropic drugs. Similarly, chapters on geriatric psychiatry and CL psychiatry are presented with basic principles, rather than describing the disorders that have already been covered in other sections or books of medical undergruate programs.

Refer the cover of the book to explore online MCQs and Clinical Cases, which we have painstakingly developed especially for you. The symbols ⓜ and ◑ in the table of contents of this book will help you identify these online resources. Besides these, you will get access to the complimentary e-book also.

I hope that you will find this book useful! If you have any suggestions or critical comments to improve the content of this book, please share them with me.

Ravi Gupta
sleepclinic.india@gmail.com
ravigupta@srhu.edu.in

Acknowledgements

Writing a book is a huge task and besides the author many other people contribute to the cause.

At first, I would like to thank THE ALMIGHTY for providing me with the idea, wisdom, patience and perseverance to complete this book.

I would also like to acknowledge the contributions of my teachers who taught me the finer aspects of Psychiatry during my postgraduate training. I can distinctly remember the contribution of faculty of Department of Psychiatry, SMS Medical College, Jaipur including Dr RK Solanki, Dr Pradeep Sharma, Dr Shiv Gautam, Dr Anil Tambi, Dr Sanjay Jain, Dr Krishna Kanwal, Dr Lalit Batra, Dr ID Gupta, Dr Alok Tyagi, Dr Suresh Gupta and Dr Paramjeet Singh. Each one of them was an expert in his area and taught me the subject with affection and patience. Though I made multiple mistakes during learning, they brought them to my notice in a non-critical manner and guided me. Whatever little I have learnt in this field, whole credit goes to them.

Some people in my life have not been my teachers directly, but they always helped and guided me in my academic endeavours. I consider them as my mentors. Dr E Mohan Das, Past President, Indian Psychiatric Society was the key person to draw my interest in biological psychiatry. He always inspired me to improve my reading habits and remain updated. This is the one reason that I could understand the Psychiatry in neurobiological terms. Dr MS Bhatia, my supervisor during PhD, carved a scientific author out of me and under his able guidance I wrote my initial manuscripts for various books as well as journals. This book had not been there, if he would not have refined my writing skills. Here, I would also like to acknowledge Dr Rajat Ray, Ex-HOD, Department of Psychiatry, All India Institute of Medical Sciences, New Delhi, and the brain behind establishing the National Drug Dependence Treatment Center, Ghaziabad. I consider myself fortunate to have his blessings, he guided me throughout this project and provided me his critical but invaluable suggestions regarding the content and design of this book.

I shall also remain thankful to Dr (Maj) Nandkishore, Past President, Indian Psychiatric Society-Central Zone, who always guided me during my journey in the academic world. My dear friend and an eminent neurologist, Dr Deepak Goel, has always been a source of support and inspiration. I shall remain indebted to them for having faith in me and encouraging me in my adademic endevours.

It is my privilege that two eminent Sleep Physicians, Dr Robert Farney and Dr Jim Walker of LDS Hospital, Salt Lake city, Utah had been my teachers and mentors in Sleep Medicine. They taught me the intricacies of Sleep Medicine and helped me to understand this complex subject. Though I spent a brief time with them, yet they left an everlasting impression on me.

I am thankful to the reviewers who spared their valuable time to review the content in this book. Without their critical suggestions, this book could not have taken present shape. Their names are appearing on the page "Reviewers".

No work can be accomplished without the help of friends. I would like to acknowledge my friends Dr Purav Kumar Midha, Dr Vaibhav Dubey, Dr Vishal Chhabra, Dr Sourav Das, Dr Ramjan Ali and Dr Mohan Dhyani who always encouraged me to work on this project and helped with their valuable suggestions time to time. Dr Mohan Dhyani, Assistant Professor, Department of Psychiatry and Sleep Clinic, Himalayan Institute of Medical Sciences, also contributed four chapters in the section of child psychiatry in this book.

It would be an injustice if I do not name the persons who supported me during my initial journey in the medical science. My teachers during the undergraduate years Dr Asha Bhargava, Dr S R Shukla, Dr S R Mittal, Dr Madhu Mathur, Dr Sanjeev Saxena, Dr Madan Mohan Agrawal, Dr Sanjay Singhal,

Dr Vijay Pathak and Dr Dharmendra Nagpal taught me not only the subjects but also the human values. My seniors Dr Abhishek Chaturvedi and Dr Ramandeep Singh Brar guided me in each and every step during this journey. My friends Dr Reetu Bachhawat, Dr Pavan Pandey, Dr Giriraj Singh Bora, Dr Mukesh Parashar, Dr Pawan Singhal, Dr Rajanish Sharma, Dr Deepak Tiwari, Dr Supriy Jain, Dr Dhruva Chawla and Dr Rajeev Upadhyay have always been a source of support. Their constructive criticisms and encouragment helped me to improve my understanding of the medical science as a subject.

I would also like to take this oportunity to express my gradtuitude to the administration of Himalayan Institute of Medical Sciences, Dehradun for allowing me to use the clinical material from the hospital as illustration in this book. I am also thankful to the editors of various journals who permitted me to use illustrations from their journals in this book.

I am delighted and thankful to have a team of wonderful people associated with me throughout this project in ELSEVIER. This project started with my discussions with Dr Renu Rawat; she helped me throughout this project and provided valuable suggestions to improve on the content and presentation. Ms Shabina Nasim contributed with her inputs at all stages of this project. Ms Nayagi Athmanathan's eye for detail contributed to the quality of the book. Mr Shravan Kumar worked really hard to give my manuscript the present shape. Ms Smruti helped me working on the digital part of this project.

Last but not least, I shall always remian thankful to my family members—my parents, my wife Dr Vibha Gupta and my daughter Anshulika. My parents always inspired and guided me. Vibha provided invaluable suggestions on the content and presentation of this book. Without her and Anshulika's emotional support this project would have been a nought.

Ravi Gupta

Reviewers

Alka Subramanyam
Sr. Assistant Professor
Department of Psychiatry
Topiwala National Medical College &
BYL Nair Charitable Hospital, Mumbai

Anil Nischal
Associate Professor
Department of Psychiatry
KGMU, Lucknow

Arshad Hussain
Associate Professor
Institute of Mental Health & Neurosciences,
Kashmir
Affiliated to Government Medical College,
Srinagar

Atul Ambekar
Additional Professor
Department of Psychiatry
All India Institute of Medical Sciences,
New Delhi

Gaurav Rajender
Assistant Professor
Department of Psychiatry
SMS Medical College, Jaipur

Kanchan Bhasin
Final year MBBS
Himalayan Institute of Medical Sciences,
Dehradun

Nikhilesh Mandal
Assistant Professor
Institute of Psychiatry,
Institute of Postgraduate Medical Education
and Research, Kolkata

Rohit Gupta
Assistant Professor
Department of Medicine
Himalayan Institute of Medical Sciences,
Dehradun

Sandeep Goyal
Professor
Department of Psychiatry
Christian Medical College,
Ludhiana

Santosh Kumar
Assistant Professor
Department of Psychiatry
Nalanda Medical College,
Patna

Vaibhav Dubey
Associate Professor
Department of Psychiatry
People's Medical College, Bhopal

Vrinda Saxena
Final year MBBS
Himalayan Institute of Medical Sciences,
Dehradun

Contents

PSYCHIATRY: EMERGING NEUROSCIENCE

1.1

Ravi Gupta

A 30-year-old male was brought with complaints of poor quality sleep, not working at home and lying in bed throughout the day for approximately 3 months. Symptoms progressed gradually over a few weeks in severity and were continuous. Along with these symptoms, the family members noticed a reduction in social interaction and personal care. Most of the times, the patient remained aloof and his language had become incomprehensible. The family members could not provide any history that would suggest any substance abuse, trauma to head, and any motor or sensory deficit. Medical and surgical history was negative. General physical examination disclosed that vital signs were within normal limits. Mental status examination disclosed signs of reduced motor activity and apathy. Considering the clinical picture, diagnosis of catatonia was made and a magnetic resonance scan of the brain was ordered. On scanning, a space-occupying lesion in the right parietal lobe was found causing the hydrocephalus (Fig. 1.1.1).

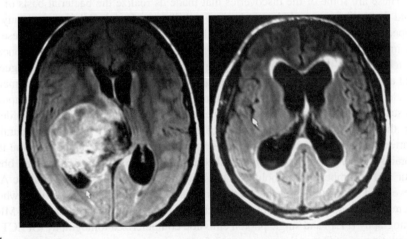

FIGURE 1.1.1

MRI scan of the brain depicting a large intracranial space occupying lesion in the right parietal lobe causing hydrocephalus.

(Source: Himalyan Hospital, Dehradun.)

1

Psychiatry, as a part of medical curriculum, has always remained an enigma for medical students. As medical students, only a few of us understand the basic concepts of psychiatry and only a selected few aspire to choose it as a profession. Some of us consider psychiatric disorders as *psychological problems or functional disorders* and unintentionally become a party to the nonscientific approaches for the diagnosis and management of patients presenting with psychiatric disorders. However, during the past 30 years, our understanding of psychiatric disorders has changed significantly and this has established psychiatry as a medical subject that deals with symptoms arising out of dysfunctional neuronal pathways. In this chapter, we will discuss some important issues that are important in understanding the pathophysiological basis of psychiatric disorders.

IS PSYCHIATRY A REAL SCIENCE?

Psychiatry refers to the study of the illnesses that manifest as change in emotions, behaviour or cognition of the sufferer. Medical illnesses originate because of pathological mechanisms in the body; likewise, pathology of the psychiatric illnesses has been traced to the brain. However, unlike brain tumours or stroke, where pathology can be viewed with naked eye, pathology in psychiatric disorders occurs at the cellular and subcellular levels. These pathological mechanisms may include, but are not limited to, altered neurotransmission owing to the change in gene expression, or receptor anomalies or disordered neuronal activation. However, understanding the pathophysiology of psychiatric disorders is still in the infantile stage and we have a long way before we fully understand the intricate mechanisms of development of psychiatric disorders.

If you recall the history of medical science, then you would be able to appreciate that nearly 150 years ago, witchcraft/magic and divine curse were considered causal to almost all medical illnesses. In 1882, Robert Koch discovered the *tuberculum bacilli*, and Alexander Fleming discovered the penicillin in 1941. These are some of the discoveries that made us realize the bacterial basis of some of the infections and that antibiotics could be synthesized to kill them. During this journey, many instruments were developed to uncover the pathophysiological basis of diseases, eg, microscope. These instruments significantly influenced our understanding that diseases and health conditions that were once considered curses or witchcrafts are medical disorders, eg, leprosy, tuberculosis, typhoid and plague, that could be diagnosed and treated. In the later part of the last century, more sophisticated instruments were developed, eg, electron microscope, electrocardiogram, electroencephalogram (EEG), computerized axial tomography scan and thermocycler. These machines expanded our vision regarding disorders.

However, the progress in neuroscience was not that rapid, especially in the behavioural part. When scientists started studying human behaviour, tools were not available that could measure the functioning of the brain. Hence, many hypothesis and theories have been proposed after keen observation of the behaviour and a number of psychological tests like Rorschach's Test and Thematic Apperception Test were developed. These tests prevailed in the psychiatry practice till late last century when high-tech machines were developed, eg, functional EEG, functional magnetic resonance imaging (f-MRI), positron emission tomography (PET) and single photon emission computerized tomography (SPECT), that could provide information regarding real-time neuronal functioning (*please refer to* Chapter 1.4). Results of the experiments that were carried out using these technological advances conveyed us the fact that all psychiatric illnesses are associated with the change in functioning of certain regions or pathways of the brain (Fig. 1.1.2). Thus, psychiatry is recognized as a branch of medical science.

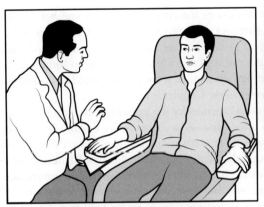 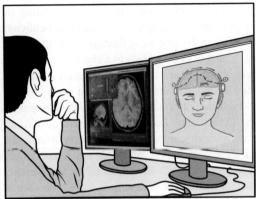

A. Psychoanalysis has not been found to have any role in management of Psychiatric disorders.

B. After few years, functional neuro-imaging could be used as a diagnostic tool for Psychiatric disorders.

FIGURE 1.1.2

Change in the diagnostic techniques in psychiatry over the years.

WHY THESE ILLNESSES ARE CALLED FUNCTIONAL?

Some people argue that psychiatric disorders are not medical disorders because we do not find any abnormality on laboratory testing. It must be remembered that the mere absence of objective evidence does not mean that a person is not having any medical disorder. Let us consider some common illness like idiopathic epilepsy or idiopathic Parkinson disease or migraine that do not show evidence of any pathology on CT or MRI. Psychiatric illnesses can be positioned in the same spectrum.

Functional disorder by no means suggests the absence of neurobiological changes; similarly, it does not suggest 'psychological' nature of illness. It just conveys that pathological changes in the organ cannot be appreciated on routine biochemical, electrophysiological, haematological or structural neuroimaging like CT or MRI. Furthermore, it denotes that the neuronal circuitry has become dysfunctional (can also be called a change in their function and thus functional) that is responsible for the symptoms. To be more precise, we can say that pathology is occurring at the level of receptor expression, receptor modulation, neurotransmitter release or inhibition, which in turn are governed by the genes and messenger systems in the neurons.

At present, the role of functional imaging techniques is limited to the research; however, with increasing understanding and stronger evidences we may expect a day when we will differentiate depression from anxiety or schizophrenia just by looking at a functional imaging scan of brain.

ROLE OF PSYCHOLOGY IN PSYCHIATRY

Many of us equate psychology with psychiatry. In fact, they cannot be compared. Psychology is a non-medical branch that focuses on the study of normal behaviour following the principles laid down by psychologists. On the other hand, psychiatry is purely a medical branch that deals with disorders, their aetiology, pathogenesis, symptomatology and treatment.

However, one must appreciate that during the process of therapy, we borrow some behavioural psychological techniques (eg, cognitive behaviour therapy; reshaping of behaviour). However, it will be unfair to say that these therapies are 'psychological', since they are based on the principle of learning, which of course leads to a change in neurocircuitry of the brain after an exposure to stimuli. Thus, these therapies are biological in nature. This is further substantiated by the fact that these therapies bring a change in the functioning of brain (*please refer to the* Chapter 9.1).

Inclusion of principles of nonmedical or paramedical faculties for the management of patients is not new in medicine. During management of coronary artery disease or diabetes, we borrow few aspects of nutritional science; during recovery from a fracture or cerebrovascular accidents, we call someone like a physiotherapist. Yet we do not equate an orthopaedist with a physiotherapist; or a cardiologist or an endocrinologist with a dietician or vice versa. I would like to emphasize that each of these streams, whether medical or nonmedical, have their own principles and their own strengths and limitations. We should not undermine any of these streams. But, it is more important to understand that one stream should not be equated with or substituted by another stream. And, lastly, as a medical student, you must understand that psychiatry is actually a neuroscience and no illness in this world is *psychological*.

DOES BEHAVIOUR HAVE A BIOLOGICAL BASIS?

Sigmund Freud (1856–1939), who had worked extensively in the field of psychology, was a physician and a neuropathologist. He studied the human behaviour extensively but could not find its physiological basis because appropriate techniques (eg, functional neuroimaging) were not available at that time. However, he was a keen observer and laid down many behavioural principles governing the human behaviour and named them psychological principles. He was convinced that the brain governs the behaviour. Still, owing to the technological limitations, dichotomy between the brain and behaviour persisted till 1960s.

Later, we learned that the mind and the brain could not be separated. Computer, if not the best, is next to the best analogy for the understanding this concept. All of us know that a computer has two components—hardware (monitor and CPU) and software. For best output, we need compatibility between the software and the hardware. If the software needs more processing than the hardware can support, you cannot run it. Similarly, if the hardware is advanced but the software is poor in quality, you cannot produce optimum output. Hence, dysfunction in either of them is sufficient to hold up the machine or to produce suboptimal results.

In case of the human brain, it may be seen as hardware, whereas cognition, emotions and behaviour can be considered software. However, this analogy is *not fool proof*. In case of computers, software and hardware are developed and assembled separately and software can be loaded on the hardware. On the contrary, in the case of brain, the software (cognition, emotions, behaviours) *continues to learn from experiences and thus it keeps changing* over time and for this to happen, adequate functioning of hardware (proper functioning of individual neuron; adequate and appropriate flow of information between neurons in a given area of brain and between different areas of brain) is of paramount importance. Thus, any change in the functioning of software of the brain (behavioural, emotional or cognitive functions) undoubtedly implies that a problem with the hardware is present. This malfunctioning can be grossly visible, eg, damage to the motherboard of the computer (*may be equated with a stroke or a tumour in the brain*), or—sometimes at the microscopic level—disrupted functions in integrated circuits (ICs) of the computer (*equated with functional dysfunctions at the cellular or subcellular levels of neurons*).

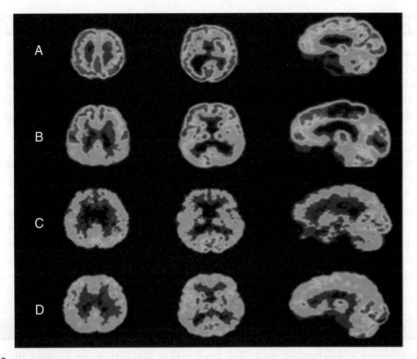

FIGURE 1.1.3

PET scan showing the functioning of different areas of the brain during a mental task.

Any damage to the hardware (dysgenesis or degeneration or damage to the brain) alters the expression of the software resulting in behavioural change akin to intellectual disability or neurocognitive disorders or behavioural and emotional symptoms. Similarly, sometimes there is no gross damage to the hardware, but just the current cannot flow properly owing to microstructural changes and this state gives rise to symptoms of mood disorders, psychotic disorders, addiction, delirium, migraine, idiopathic epilepsy and idiopathic Parkinson disease (Fig. 1.1.3).

PSYCHIATRIC DISORDERS: ROLE OF GENES

Psychiatric disorders often run in families. First-degree relatives are at a higher risk for having the illness than the general population. Twin studies show that monozygotic twins have higher chances of development of disorders as compared to dizygotic twins. In essence, these disorders have a genetic basis. However, like hypertension, diabetes or coronary artery disease, these disorders also show multifactorial inheritance. This is one reason why only some members of the family are affected or at other times few generations are spared in a family with psychiatric disorders. This makes the genetics an important branch of psychiatry and also favours the biological basis of the illnesses.

MISCONCEPTIONS ABOUT "PSYCHOLOGICAL" ORIGIN OF SYMPTOMS

Some medical professionals consider that when they are not able to find any 'organic' cause for medical illness in any patient, then the patient should be sent for a psychiatrist's opinion. On the other hand, few professionals think that a patient having been diagnosed of any 'organic' disorder cannot suffer from any psychiatric ailment. Actually, both these are extreme views and unfortunately none of them stands true. From the discussion so far, we know that *psychiatric disorders are actually 'organic'*. We must also appreciate the fact that any change occurring in the body during medical illness may influence the neurotransmission and can initiate a psychiatric disorder.

It must be remembered that behavioural problems emerging during a medical disorder may represent a psychiatric disorder. For example, sad mood during the course of tuberculosis may be a symptom of depression. Similarly, when a symptom for a given medical illness occurs in excess of what is expected out of the pathophysiological findings, it may represent a psychiatric illness. A patient with rheumatoid arthritis may keep complaining of pain despite radiological and serological improvement in the arthritis. In this case, persistent pain could represent a psychiatric illness. However, symptoms must be sufficiently severe and last for optimal duration to qualify for the diagnosis of psychiatric illness, otherwise psychiatric disorders cannot be diagnosed. *In other words, psychiatric disorders are not the diagnosis of exclusion.*

DICHOTOMY OF NEUROLOGY AND PSYCHIATRY

This is an interesting and debatable issue. You must realize that dichotomy is more theoretical than practical. Essentially, both the functions are governed by the same organ—the brain. Earlier *psychiatry* and *neurology* were one discipline and were taught as a single branch of medicine.

With time, scientists started finding cause for neurological illness, as they were more conspicuous—damage of certain areas/neurons and modalities to objectively assess them (microscope) were available. On the other hand, unfortunately, psychological theories dominated psychiatry in the absence of functional neuroimaging techniques and Psychiatry was left to be considered closer to psychology than to neuroscience. A major breakthrough came when functional imaging techniques had started depicting that psychiatric symptoms *were* actually related to the altered brain functioning. We also know that neurological illnesses have behavioural manifestations and psychiatric disorders have at least subtle neurological dysfunction. Thus, this dichotomy is more artificial than natural.

FUTURE OF PSYCHIATRY

Today's psychiatry may be equated with behavioural neurology. With the advancement of knowledge, it has been expanded and many subspecialties have developed within psychiatry (Table 1.1.1).

Table 1.1.1 Subspecialties in Psychiatry

Child and adolescent psychiatry[a]	Headache medicine
General adult psychiatry	Forensic psychiatry
Geriatric psychiatry[a]	Neuropsychopharmacology
Addiction medicine[a]	Psychiatry genetics
Consultation liaison psychiatry	Psychiatric epidemiology
Psychosomatic medicine	Neuropsychiatry
Sleep medicine	Perinatal psychiatry

[a]In these subspecialties, DM courses are available at some of the Indian institutes.

SUMMARY

- Psychiatry is an expending field of neuroscience.
- All psychiatric disorders have neurobiological basis.
- Psychiatry can be equated with behavioural neurology.
- Psychiatry is an expanding field with the development of many subspecialties.
- Psychiatry is a medical branch that cannot be equated to psychology.

HISTORY TAKING AND EXAMINATION OF A PSYCHIATRIC PATIENT

1.2

Ravi Gupta

Medical history is the information that is obtained from a patient or his/her informants regarding his/her illness. It helps in reaching to a diagnosis and guides management. Obtaining an informative history requires a good fund of knowledge and clinical skills. One of the basic and important clinical skills is the establishment of rapport with the patient and his/her family members so that intricate personal issues may be unfolded. For this, one requires to encompass the art of communication. Thus, it is a science that runs itself on the wheel of an art.

History taking is important in all streams of medical science where one need to deal with a patient, eg, medicine, surgery, obstetrics. However, it becomes more important in neuropsychiatric disorders where objective tests are either not available or have limitations and thus contribute little to substantiate or corroborate the information obtained during history taking. Therefore, you should always spend ample time in obtaining history while dealing with a patient of neurological or psychiatric disorder.

PREREQUISITES OF HISTORY TAKING

These prerequisites are not exclusive to the psychiatry practice but apply to practice of any branch of medical science.

RAPPORT

As we have already discussed, informative history can only be obtained after establishing a rapport with the informants and patient. Rapport can be established by asking few questions about the patient or his/her family. However, it is not as easy as it appears because you are in the process of making a bond with a stranger and you want him/her to divulge his/her personal information and that too in a short time. Therefore, you must look comfortable, patient and interested in understanding and solving patient's problems. Impatient gestures and movements must be best avoided, and the stance should be positive and empathetic.

EYE CONTACT

Whether to look directly in a patient's eye during history taking and mental status examination is a controversial issue. Some authorities suggest that direct gaze may be perceived offensive by the patient, especially females, and it is best to look just below the eyes of the patient. However, you may choose to not to keep your gaze fixed at any particular body part, but to maintain a comfortable eye contact.

SETTING

The place that you offer to the patient and his/her family members (informants) to sit with you is also important. It is better to avoid frequent intrusion of any unwanted person and place must be large enough to accommodate you, patient and informants with optimal amount of lighting, ventilation, temperature and furniture.

PRIVACY

Though the privacy must be respected in all medical branches, it becomes more important when as a psychiatrist you are dealing with behavioural and emotional symptoms. Patients often have issues that they do not want to disclose to anybody except the clinician, eg, sexual orientation, sexual encounters and information regarding substance abuse. Similarly, symptoms in psychiatric illness are mainly behavioural, and patient or the informants may not want to disclose the behavioural aberrations to anybody else except the clinician. It is important to respect these feelings and maintain the confidentiality.

TAKING NOTES

While taking the history, it is advisable not to rely solely on your memory. It is better to take written notes. This will help you in probing deeply into every complaint of the patient at the time of initial examination as well as help in maintaining the record. Future progress can also be tracked by measuring the improvement of target symptoms on subsequent visits. Should any new symptom emerge during the therapy, it provides a clue to the adverse effects of the drugs or development of a new illness. It also helps in medico-legal cases.

ELEMENTS OF THE HISTORY

History is always taken in a particular sequence, so as to ensure that any information does not get missed. Though there are many schools of thoughts and many performas, we are providing one that is easy to remember and is followed at most of the places. The points to be covered and their order should be as follows:

1. Details of informants
2. Sociodemographic data
3. Presenting complaints with duration
4. (A) Predisposing, precipitating and perpetuating factors, if any (for the illness since onset),
   (B) aggravating and relieving factors (for the present episode)
5. Onset: abrupt/acute/gradual (for present episode)
6. Course: progressive/stable/remitting/relapsing-remitting (since onset of illness)
7. Presence of symptoms: continuous/intermittent (for present episode)

8. History of present illness:
   (i) details of the presenting complaints
   (ii) negative history
9. History of change in personal, social and occupational functioning due to symptoms
10. Past history of psychiatric and/or medical illness
11. Treatment history:
    (i) treatment taken with duration
    (ii) compliance of patient
    (iii) any adverse effect with the drugs
    (iv) response to therapy
12. Family history: family members, interpersonal relationships, social network, patient's interaction with network (quantitatively and qualitatively), instrumental support, perceived support, family history of any illness
13. Developmental history
14. Psychosexual history
15. Premorbid personality

1. DETAILS OF INFORMANT

It is of vital importance to keep the details (eg, name, age and relationship with the patient) of the informant. In clinical settings, a person that has witnessed a patient for sufficiently long period, who stays with the patient, who himself/herself 'appears' to be of sound mind, and who 'appears' interested in patient's welfare is considered a reliable informant. Since it is not easy to check the trustworthiness of accompanying person, the word 'appears' has been used in last two criteria.

Whenever the information mismatches grossly with the mental status of the patient, such remark must be made in the history sheet in such a way that it cannot be tempered. In such cases, you may defer your diagnosis or keep the patient under observation till the final diagnosis is made or call another informant.

Another important thing to consider is the reliability of the informant. In some instances, patients are not able to provide reliable information. For example, a person with paranoid delusion may not trust you and thus remains guarded. A person with substance abuse may try to minimize the amount and duration of the substance or may try to omit some of the facts. A person with neurocognitive disorder may not be able to provide adequate information owing to cognitive dysfunction. Since, the symptoms of psychiatric disorders are behavioural, their expression may be manipulated. Thus, an alleged psychiatric patient may appear completely normal on cross-sectional examination or vice versa. In the circumstances like these, you may require parallel information from the family member or a friend (informant) and his/her reliability must be ascertained (vide infra).

VIGNETTE

A violent patient was brought in the clinic by three informants. The patient was tied in ropes; he was shouting at his informants and was abusing them. He was accusing that they wanted him to be declared lunatic to snatch his property. The informants asked the psychiatrist for help and gave the history of sudden onset of progressive illness since past 7 days. On brief history and examination, psychiatrist found discrepancies between the history and mental status examination. He asked the supporting staff to untie the patient, offered him some water and talked to him in a separate room. Even now, he could not elicit any signs of illness except paranoid ideas against his informants who happened to be his brothers.

Due to gross mismatch in history and examination, he admitted the patient under observation and asked the informants to call some other informant, especially one who patient wanted to come. On subsequent examinations and other informants' clues, it became clear that patient was not ill and his account of circumstances was true.

2. SOCIODEMOGRAPHIC DATA

This is similar to the data that we gather during history taking in other branches. Patient's name, father's/mother's name, age, sex, address, marital status, monthly family income, occupation must be noted. Each of these elements is important and helps us in the process of either diagnosis or management.

Name gives an identity to the patient so that his/her file can be tracked from the record. Calling a patient with his/her name rather than 'bed number so and so' helps in establishment of rapport.

Age helps in convergence of the diagnosis since most of the diseases start at a certain time periods in a person's life. For example, cognitive impairment since birth is found in intellectual disability, while its occurrence after a period of normal development is seen in autistic spectrum disorders, encephalopathy and Creutzfeldt–Jakob disease. If it occurs in older age, it can best be described as neurocognitive disorder. Table 1.2.1 deciphers the age of onset for common psychiatric ailments. Moreover, it also suggests which other illness to be looked for that may help in explaining the disease itself or provides a useful clue to the management.

Clue regarding the diagnosis can be found from gender as prevalence may differ

Table 1.2.1 Age of Onset of Some Disorders[a]

Age of Onset	Illness
Infancy to early childhood	Intellectual disability Autistic spectrum disorders Enuresis Specific learning disorders ADHD Epilepsy Metabolic storage diseases
Adolescence	Substance use disorders Sexual disorders Mood disorders Schizophrenia Anxiety spectrum disorders Trauma to CNS Cerebral infections Hypothyroidism
Early adulthood	Mood disorders Schizophrenia Cerebrovascular disorders Multiple sclerosis
Late adulthood	Early onset dementia Intracranial tumours
Elderly	Neurodegenerative disorders, eg, Parkinsonism, Alzheimer disease

[a]*These are approximate age of onset, which can vary at times in certain cases. Remember biology always has exceptions to the rule.*

across genders. While migraine, tension type headache, depression, conversion disorders, somatic symptoms disorders, fibromyalgia, restless legs syndrome and insomnia are more common among females; disorders like drug abuse, attention deficit hyperactivity disorder (ADHD), disruptive behaviour and obstructive sleep apnoea are more frequent among males. Few symptoms, eg, premature ejaculation, nocturnal emission are found only in men.

Monthly family income provides a clue regarding affordability of the treatment and may help in planning the treatment especially when the person is not a beneficiary of the medical insurance. Similarly, occupation not only gives a clue regarding person's social and educational background but also suggests workplace related factors that contribute in development of pathology, eg, persons working in shifts with insomnia may actually have the shift worker's disorder; what appears as somatic symptoms disorder could be a consequence of insufficient sleep owing to shift work.

3. PRESENTING COMPLAINTS

These are those symptoms with which the patient presents to the physician. There are two methods for noting the complaints. First, according to the severity: most severe complaints are asked first followed by complaints with lesser concern. This is a good method for ascertainment of treatment as more troublesome symptoms may be targeted in the initial period to provide quick relief. However, this approach does not disclose evolution of the disease and thus comorbidities may be missed that may be of serious concern. Second approach of recording the complaints follows chronology of the appearance of symptoms: In this method we try to arrange the symptoms chronologically, ie, symptom that appeared first should be first, and so on. It provides the sequelae of development of symptoms and thus gives an idea regarding the pathophysiology of illness. This approach leads to the diagnosis.

Examples of these approaches are illustrated in Table 1.2.2.

Thus, the history should be obtained in chronological order to reach to a diagnosis, but while planning the management, severity of the symptoms *that fits the diagnosis* should be kept in mind. In the case depicted in Table 1.2.2, after making the diagnosis of delirium, antipsychotics may be started to address most severe symptom, ie, hyperactivity.

It is important to note that presenting complaints should be asked from the patient as well from the informant. So you will be having two versions of the complaints. Since, you are dealing with the behavioural complaints, it is essential to note that both versions (patient's as well as informant's) should be seen in view of the findings of the mental status examination and should be considered complimentary rather than contradictory.

Table 1.2.2 Diagnosis Depends Upon How you Take the History

According to Severity	Chronological Order
Talks to self	Weakness
Hearing voices	Weight gain
Violent behaviour	Poor appetite
Abusive sometimes	Decreased sleep
Abnormal talks	Disordered sleep
Decreased sleep	Abusive at times
Disordered sleep	Hearing voices
Weakness	Talks to self
Poor appetite	Abnormal talks
Weight gain	Violent behaviour
Probable diagnosis:	*Probable diagnosis:*
Psychotic episode	Delirium secondary to CHF

4. PREDISPOSING, PRECIPITATING AND PERPETUATING FACTORS

It is necessary to understand the difference between predisposing, precipitating and perpetuating factors since each of these factors may guide us in planning the treatment and estimation of prognosis. However, psychiatric disorders may start de novo and these factors may not be identified.

Predisposing factors are those characteristics of a person that he/she is born with, ie, the genetic constitution. Since almost all psychiatric disorders follow multifactorial inheritance, family history of the disorder or in other words, shared gene pool predisposes a person to develop a given illness. Though we have mentioned predisposing factors here for the sake of better understanding, they are usually recorded while taking family history.

Precipitating factors are those conditions that lead to decompensation of the physiological milieu and start the illness. In cases of trauma and stress-related disorders, a stress may act as a precipitating factor; in other cases illness may be precipitated by ingestion of a drug or a substance of abuse or a medical illness. However, stress and traumatic events are ubiquitous and everybody is exposed to them. In psychiatric cases especially, trauma and stress are perhaps given undue importance. Some of us attribute every psychiatric disorder to stress; however, it is practically impossible to see any patient (suffering from any illness whether medical, surgical or psychiatric) who has not suffered any stress during past few days (*please refer to unresolved issues in chapter 3.6*).

Perpetuating factors are those elements that maintain the illness, once it has started. Sometimes patient may have more than one factor and at times they have synergistic effect, eg, hunger can precipitate a migraine episode and hot environment and continuing hunger may perpetuate it.

While planning a treatment, physician must clearly explain to family members that timely identification and prevention of precipitating factors is of paramount importance. It would reduce the frequency of illness and thus would make it amenable to treatment. Avoidance of perpetuating factors would have same effect.

By having experience in the history taking in medicine and surgery, you must already be familiar with aggravating and relieving factors. They should also be asked in certain cases like headache, delirium and sleep apnoea.

5. ONSET OF ILLNESS

Onset of illness should be determined with as certainty as possible because it provides clue regarding not only the aetiology but also towards prognosis. An illness can start in one of the three modes—abruptly, acutely or gradually. Though there are no strict guidelines for the three terms, for the sake of understanding, abrupt signifies development of full-blown symptoms within 48 h from the period of normalcy; acute onset suggests that symptom reached to peak in the span of 2–7 days; and gradual onset denotes appearance of full-blown illness over weeks.

Abrupt onset is *usually* seen after substance use (intoxication or withdrawal) or it may be medication-induced or may be associated with medical morbidity. However, most of the psychiatric disorders that appear de novo have acute and gradual onset, as they require recruitment of a number of brain areas.

6. COURSE OF ILLNESS

After onset of illness, it may run one of the following course—remitting, progressive, stable or relapsing-remitting (Fig. 1.2.1). Moreover, remission may either be complete or may be associated with residual illness. As a result, patient may achieve baseline functioning or may suffer deterioration in functioning.

However, during history of present episode, it is sufficient to chart it on one of the three modes: remitting, progressive or stable since other factors require information of past episodes. Remitting course may be seen when the patient has a disorder that naturally runs a short course, eg, dissociative disorder, conversion disorder; or that patient has been brought after a long time has been elapsed since the onset of illness or has been given some treatment before seeking your consultation.

Progressive course depicts increment of underlying pathology, which may be related to the disease process or inadequate care of patient. It may be reported if patient is brought within few days while the disease was evolving. In some circumstances, it also suggests substance intoxication or substance withdrawal since withdrawal symptoms aggravate for few days. Similarly, stable course can be seen after many episodes as in long-standing schizophrenia, persistent depressive disorder (when the maximal damage has occurred and there is no room for more damage); or in cases of partial response to the drugs if the patient has been treated.

7. NATURE OF ILLNESS

During the present episode (ie, most recent symptomatic period), symptoms may be continuous or may fluctuate in severity. Continuous illness in the present episode suggests persistent underlying pathology, eg, schizophrenia, episode of mania, intracranial space occupying lesions or encephalopathy.

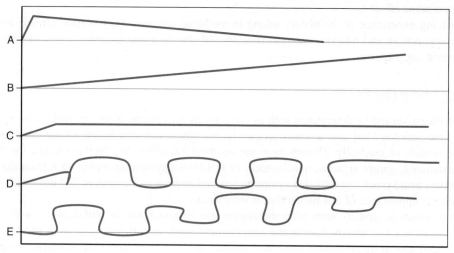

FIGURE 1.2.1

Various courses that a disease may follow.

Fluctuating severity of illness is unusual in primary psychiatric illness except in cyclothymia, ultrarapid cycling mood disorder, borderline personality disorders, dissociative disorders, epilepsy, third ventricular tumours with ball valve mechanisms, substance-induced disorders with repeated substance consumption, and repeated cerebrovascular events, to name a few.

8. HISTORY OF PRESENT ILLNESS

It is the heart of the information gathering process as it gives you finer details regarding the nature of symptoms, points towards the underlying aetiology, helps in assessment of severity of each symptom and narrows down the differential diagnosis for focused clinical and laboratory examination.

By the time you reach this point, you often have a broad idea regarding possible diagnosis; therefore, you must probe into each symptom thoroughly and try to establish what you would like to examine during the physical and mental status examination. However, you should not be overenthusiastic regarding possible diagnosis as it may tunnel your vision and limit the probability of reaching to the correct diagnosis.

For example, if complaints of 'suspicious of spouse's character' are present, its onset, development, course, acting on the belief must be established by proxy. Informants should be asked regarding patients' reaction when they tried to contradict his/her false belief; enquire about behavioural changes in the patient while dealing with spouse and other family members; and lastly, any association with external factors (eg, behaviour becomes more problematic when spouse talks to person of opposite sex, or after substance use by the patient). This helps in differentiation of delusion from an idea, assesses its severity (firmer the belief, more severe is the illness) and it's emotional valence for the patient. Similarly, when a patient presents with some hallucinatory behaviour, one must ask for the timing of appearance of hallucinations, circumstances that aggravate the hallucinations, persistence of hallucinations and patient's apparent response to hallucinations.

Similarly, in a person with violent behaviour or irritability, it is imperative to ask about the precipitating factors, whether it occurs in response to internal (patient-related factors that may not be known to informants) or external stimuli, what the patient does during the episode, duration of each episode, reaction of patient once the episode lasts, etc. This may help to differentiate between simple partial seizure, irritability seen in depression, excitement seen in schizophrenia, manic irritability, irritability secondary to a substance abuse and impulse control disorder.

We have presented few examples of dissecting the information that you should gather for some of the abnormal behaviours. However, behaviour varies from time to time and from person to person and it is not possible to provide what should be asked for every such behaviour. These are some of the points that you need to ask; however, there may be many more depending upon the complaints and circumstances of the patient. You will learn them with experience. In addition to experience, you need to improve your fund of knowledge.

Negative history should be mentioned to narrow down the diagnostic possibilities that you have reached so far! A good negative history not only guides you to the correct diagnosis but also makes the foundation for physical and mental status examination.

Note: There is no substitute for the fund of knowledge. A good psychiatrist should have working knowledge of medical and neurological disorders in addition to psychiatry.

9. CHANGES IN THE PATIENT'S FUNCTIONING DUE TO SYMPTOMS

Remember, psychiatric symptoms are largely behavioural and expression of behaviour occurs over a spectrum. A behaviour that is considered normal in one circumstance may be abnormal in another. Besides qualitative dimension, behaviour also has a quantitative aspect. Hence, just the abnormal behaviour may not call for the treatment, unless this symptom is imposing any interference with the patient's personal, social or occupational life. To make it clearer, a number of people may be categorized as having 'reserved nature'. If the person is doing well in all three spheres—social, occupational and personal he/she may not need any treatment. Hence, clinician must always ask if the symptoms are interfering with the patient's functioning.

10. PAST HISTORY OF PSYCHIATRIC OR MEDICAL ILLNESS

Past history is an integral part of the diagnostic process. It not only helps in establishing the diagnosis, but also guides you regarding the prognosis and future course of illness. Besides that, it also assists you in determining the duration of treatment and helps you to pick the best medication. For example, a patient who is presenting with the symptoms of depression will be diagnosed as recurrent depression, if there is a history of at least one depressive episode in past. However, the diagnosis will change to bipolar disorder if manic episodes can be established in past. Depressive symptoms arising in a patient with congestive heart failure (CHF) may indicate failing heart and in Parkinson disease patient may indicate progression of this neurodegenerative illness.

11. TREATMENT HISTORY

It must be remembered that patients may have selective response, to a class of drugs (eg, better to selective serotonin reuptake inhibitor (SSRI) as compared to serotonin and norepinephrine reuptake inhibitor (SNRI) or towards one molecule from a class of drugs (eg, better response with fluoxetine as compared to sertraline). Second, some patients may not feel comfortable with one molecule but at the same time, may tolerate another molecule in a better manner. For example, a patient with mania may not like valproate owing to certain reasons (eg, size of the tablet) but may not hesitate to take lithium. Third, a patient may not be compliant to one drug owing to adverse effects but may show better compliance to another because of its better side-effect profile or therapeutic response. Hence, treatment history must always be clarified in detail so as to plan your future course of action. Special attention must be given to response of the molecule, treatment emergent adverse effects, doses, duration of treatment and factors associated with compliance in the past. Treatment history also helps in choosing the route of drug. Depot preparations may be prescribed to a person who is responding well to a drug, still is noncompliant secondary to disease factors (Table 1.2.3).

12. FAMILY HISTORY AND AVAILABLE SUPPORT

As already mentioned in the earlier chapter (Chapter 1.1) that psychiatric illnesses have a genetic origin and often run in families. Hence, it is important to ask about the family members that might be affected from psychiatric illness. This genetic loading in a patient increases the chances of recurring episodes as well as that of poor response to treatment. Besides that, certain unusual responses to the treatment

Table 1.2.3 How Treatment History Helps in Management

Condition	Response
Good response to molecule A	Start with the same molecule in future episodes
Poor compliance due to adverse effects with molecule A	**Approach 1:** Weigh risk-benefit ratio; explain benefits of continuing A to the patient; use correctives to reduce adverse effects **Approach 2:** Try another molecule and watch for adverse effects
Poor compliance due to disease-related factors	Plan depot preparation; use liquid preparation of the drug

are more likely to appear if a family member is having a history of a particular psychiatric disorder. For example, in a patient with major depressive disorder, who has the family history of bipolar disorder, antidepressants may induce manic episode.

Not only the diagnosis, but the family history also guides to the treatment. It has been found that response to a given drug often runs in families. In other words, a patient with depression is more likely to respond to SSRI, if his/her father had same illness and responded well to SSRIs.

Thirdly, family history gives you an idea about ongoing stress (when we ask about the interpersonal relationships of family members), and instrumental support (financial and physical support offered by the family members). This information provides clues for the adequate planning of treatment; eg, it helps to decide on the issues like medication to be prescribed (based upon cost; seeking medical help in case of adverse effects), route of doses (oral, daily pills vs. long-acting depot injections). Any interpersonal distress is to be addressed during the therapy since it may interfere with the patient's perception of the improvement in symptoms. Similarly, patients with poor instrumental support may require assistance during the therapy and may need to be hospitalized.

You should also enquire regarding patient's interaction with the available social network (quantitatively and qualitatively), as it tells us about the patient's perception of illness and you may plan to use the available social resources in the therapy, eg, a substance-user having friends who are football players may be motivated to join the group and he may be encouraged to learn to enjoy the 'kick' out of the game rather than that of substance use.

It is best to depict the information in a pedigree chart.

13. PERSONAL HISTORY

Developmental history is important while you are dealing with patients in paediatrics, psychiatry and neurology. It includes perinatal history, postnatal history and developmental milestones (including motor, sensory and behavioural). Behaviour at school is an important issue that needs to be ascertained. It is important because patients having neurodevelopmental disorder may have a different expression of symptoms during adulthood. Neurodevelopmental problems are the cause of concern, especially when you are working in a child psychiatry unit.

Psychosexual history is an important part of the medical and psychiatric history. One must ask about the sexuality, sexual orientation, sexual preferences, encounters, sexual activity, etc. In India, where the sexual misconceptions are prevalent, one must try to gather the information regarding issues like 'dhat' discharge, and deviation of penis. Patients having these misconceptions may be distressed that can be mistaken for depression or another psychiatric disorder. In addition, these problems may sometimes be related to other disorders, eg, other diabetes mellitus, Parkinson disease, obstructive sleep apnoea or depression. At other times, they may be related to the treatment (antipsychotics may reduce libido by inducing hyperprolactinaemia and antidepressants may cause delayed ejaculation or erectile dysfunction).

14. PREMORBID PERSONALITY

Patient's personality traits before emergence of psychiatric illness must be explored. Undoubtedly, a change in 'personality' depicts onset of a psychiatric illness. Many a times, disease presentation may vary from the classical clinical picture depending upon the personality traits, eg, depression may manifest as irritability in a hyperthymic patient. Personality traits sometimes convert into a disorder and can be the cause of concern.

Major areas that are to be explored include interpersonal relationship, functioning at the workplace, participation in family and community activities, patient's perception of people around him/her, how does he/she usually feels (temperament), what does other people opine about him/her *(please refer to chapter 3.8)*.

WHAT DO WE CONCLUDE?

Thus, we have seen that like any other medical or surgical branch, history is very important in psychiatry practice as well. A good history can unfold the mystery of the patient's abnormal behaviour; however, to obtain a good history, you must have adequate knowledge. Many disorders may be excluded based upon the history only, thus reducing the time spent in examination and minimizing the laboratory investigations. Furthermore, a good history helps you in planning the treatment and improves the compliance.

EXAMINATION OF THE PATIENT

We have covered the part of history taking at length because history in psychiatry is slightly different. However, we will abbreviate the part of examination because you can read it from any book describing the medical examination.

Examination of the patient starts with general physical examination, eg, pulse rate, blood pressure, respiratory rate, temperature and conjunctival examination. Individual system may be examined depending upon the presenting complaints.

General physical examination starts right when the patient enters your room. Check for his/her *attire, gait, posture, facial expressions, nonverbal behaviour, behaviour with other persons* in your room, eg, yourself, other staff members and family members. Poor self-care may be seen during depression, dementia, delirium, schizophrenia and substance intoxication to name a few. On the other hand, histrionic patients and those with manic episode may present with flamboyant clothing. Patient with depression or Parkinson disease may have slow gait, short steps; those with stroke show hemiplegic gait; cerebellar disorders and peripheral sensory neuropathy may present with ataxic gait; patients having anxiety or akathisia may be pacing. One must also notice for abnormal motor activity, eg, tremors and dyskinesia. This may help you in arriving to a diagnosis and focusing your interview with the patient. While noting the behaviour with yourself and other persons in the room, you have a chance to examine social judgment of the patient. While you start the dialogue with him/her, you can examine the rapport.

Rapport can be established with the patients by asking few biographical questions. Rapport simply means that you and your patient are working on the same wavelength. In some cases, patient is secretive, does not want to share his/her problem and does not help you in the examination. This can be seen in delirium, paranoid delusions or when patient does not trust you. In some cases, patients open up after some difficulty, eg, when a person seeks help for the sexual problem or addiction while in some other cases, patient may appear 'open' at first look. This can be seen in situation of mania, histrionic personality and disinhibited states. You should make a note of it.

TESTING OF HIGHER MENTAL FUNCTIONS

First to be assessed is the *consciousness* of the patient. It is very difficult to define consciousness, but it can be considered as the person's ability to be aware and respond to the environment appropriately. You may get an idea about the level of consciousness after communicating with the person for some time. After checking the consciousness, you should check the *orientation* of the person towards to environment, eg, time, place and person. While doing this, you must make sure that you ask the right question, eg, if you ask a person 'what time is it?' when he/she is placed in a room which does not have any window opening to the outside (as happens in most of the ICUs), he/she may not provide you the correct response. The better way is to first ask him/her look outside the window, get an idea of light and then reply. Similarly, if you ask 'which place are you in?' and you are expecting your hospital's name from a person who has been brought in a state of altered consciousness, you are making a mistake. Better to ask him/her 'looking at this place, where do you think are you?' Similarly, while checking the orientation to person, if the patient is able to recognize that you are a medical professional it is enough. Then his/her preparedness for the objective testing must be assessed otherwise you will get wrong interpretation.

You may get a fair idea about *attention and concentration* while you are talking to the patient. Any dysfunction in these modalities will present as confusion and incoherence. Objectively they can be tested by requesting to count numbers (forward and/or backward), or to make him utter the names of weekdays or months (either forward or backward). To make it more complex, you may use serial subtraction test (100 – 7 or 20 – 3) or use digit span test. While interpreting the results of these tests, you must be careful not to misinterpret it. A wrong calculation may suggest dyscalculia with normal concentration, provided that the patient sticks to the number serially (eg, 100, 93, 89, 83, 75). Care must be taken to consider the number of wrong responses. If attention and concentration are wandering, further testing of higher mental functions may be omitted.

Next to examine is *memory*. We examine working memory (digit span test and serial subtraction test both can also be used to examine working memory), short-term memory (what did the patient had last night, who came to visit him last day) and long-term memory (biographical and event related).

While examining memory, you should also determine if there is a problem in registration (patient not able to repeat the digit or word immediately after it was presented to him/her) or a problem in recall (registration is normal, but forgets after some time). For this, you may present with three unrelated words (three words recall test), eg, apple, cloud and money with the cues. Cue may be a short description of the object and it has to be presented with the word.

> **Physician:** I am going to present you three words. I would like you to memorize them. I will ask you all these after a while. Are you ready?
> **Patient:** OK!
> **Physician:** First word is 'apple'. It is a red fruit that most of us like. Would you please repeat the word?

Patient: Apple.

Physician: OK! Now I will present you with another word.

If a problem in non-cued recall is found, patient may be presented with cues (same as provided earlier) and one should see how many words the person can recall with cues.

Physician: You were able to tell me two words correctly. Now I will give you a clue regarding third word. It was an object that often comes with chair.

Three words recall test also examines immediate and short-term memory. After memory, we check for the *abstraction and reasoning*. Abstraction is the ability of a person to divide the whole information in small pieces and then join the facts from all the pieces to plan an appropriate response. Some of the authors suggest that abstraction can be judged by asking the proverbs, eg, 'what do you mean by "birds with same feathers?"' However, others opine that proverb testing is not adequate for two reasons: first, these proverbs have linguistic and cultural barriers and to discern the meaning the physician and the patients should have similar knowledge of language and cultural issues. Second, if the memory is intact and the person is already familiar with the proverb in question, he/she might provide spuriously correct response. Instead, we can use the similarities and dissimilarities to check ability to abstraction and reasoning. For example: you may ask what is the similarity between a bus and an airplane. Depending upon the fund of knowledge and abstraction ability of the subject you may expect a variety of replies—'both are modes of transport', 'people go from one place to other using these modes', 'both are run by the motor and fuel', 'both have engines that converts the energy from fuel to mechanical force', and so on. You can use the same clues to check for dissimilarities and again, depending upon the fund of knowledge and abstraction ability you may get a variety of responses—'one uses the principle of thrust and aerodynamics while other works on mechanical transmission', 'plane can accommodate more passengers as compared to bus', 'plane is expensive while bus is less expensive', etc.

Next in this sequence, the *judgment* is tested. Judgment can be defined as an ability to choose one option in the conflicting situation. A good judgment goes with the morally and socially acceptable norms. For example, it is normal to exchange the greetings when you meet somebody and it tests social judgment. In addition to exchange of greetings you may also notice the body language of the patient and decide whether it is appropriate to the context to substantiate your comment on social judgment. Test judgment may be recorded by asking hypothetical questions, e.g., 'what would you do if you find a purse having a currency of 5000 outside a shop?' Please remember that the response depends not only on the morality of the subject, but also by the circumstances and social norms.

Then, one should check for *fund of knowledge*. This can be judged in the professional, residential and social background of a person. A farmer, who does not have access to newspapers or mass media may not be knowing what is happening in Germany but may be well aware of the persons who have important role to play in the local community and what all does he require for getting good crop. On the contrary, another person having white-collar job in a multinational company may be oblivious of these facts.

Lastly, we check for the *insight*. It means ability to appreciate one's condition. Absence of insight is called anosognosia. In the neurology practice, it is seen in patients having right parietal lesion. However, many patients without the apparent damage to this area also lack insight; this is seen in a variety of conditions— psychosis, neurocognitive disorders, delirium, substance use disorder and intoxication. It is not exclusive to the psychiatric disorders and may be seen among other patients as well, eg, those with surgical disorders, cardiac disorders and sleep disorders. One of the factors that influences insight is the knowledge regarding the illness, its symptoms and consequences. When a person does not have the knowledge regarding the illness, he/she lacks the insight. This should be taken into consideration. Considering these issues, you should refrain from diagnosing psychosis just because a person does not have insight.

TESTING OF MENTAL STATUS

Once we are sure that higher mental functions are optimal, we start looking for other areas that reflect the mental state. It must be noticed here that the comments that you make on the following mental faculties should be made at the end of the interview when you have spent sufficient time with the patient. If you examine these areas cross-sectionally, you may draw wrong conclusions.

We have already discussed about the examination and clues from appearance of patient, establishment of *rapport* and *motor activity*. You should then examine whether the patient initiates and maintains the eye contact. It is a part of rapport building. Poor *eye contact* is seen in disinterested patient, suspicious patient, depressed patient, patient with autism spectrum disorder and one that has compromised higher mental functions. Similarly, guarded and suspicious patients may occasionally give piercing looks, so as the violent patient, but they may not like to maintain the eye contact. Patients with ADHD and anxiety are able to initiate the eye contact but are not able to sustain it.

You should pay attention to *speech* of the patient. In medical literature speech does not refer to 'ability to speak'; rather it refers to ability to communicate, which can be verbal as well as nonverbal. Thus, aphonia and mutism are not disorders of speech, while the aphasia is. When one communicates, he/she uses words and gestures. Some people speak too much to the level that you may not be able to stop them (pressure of speech), while some are careful while using the words. All these factors should be noticed in addition to loudness of the voice with reference to the context, emotional inflictions and pauses used while communicating (prosody). Subjects with anxiety and mania may have high pressure and high volume. On the other hand, patients with Parkinson disease and depression may present with low pressure (delay in communicating, long pauses and short replies), low volume and absence of prosody. Extent of *vocabulary* must be examined. It may be limited in a person who is not familiar with the language. Limited vocabulary may be seen in persons with specific learning disorders and intellectual disability. Loss of vocabulary is a feature of neurocognitive disorders also. A person with Broca's aphasia or deaf child may use only the gestures while a person with global aphasia will not communicate by any means—verbal, gestural as well as written.

During the examination, we also take note of *emotions* of the examinee. They should be examined cross-sectionally during the course of interview (*affect*). Range of emotions (anger, pride, joy, anxiety, grief) and their depth (whether he/she appeared as happy as he/she should be when you discussed about his/her achievements) should be noted. Persons with neurocognitive disorders or catatonia or severe depression may have reduced range and depth of emotions. Patients with catatonia and Parkinson disease may be apathetic and indifferent. Their appropriateness to the context should be examined (one started crying when you talked about the success of his son). Predominant emotions that you have observed during the course of interview are known as affect, eg, most of the time person appeared anxious so the affect is anxious. Then patient should be asked about the mood. Contrary to the affect, *mood* is persistent and pervasive emotional tone that influences a person's life. So you may ask 'how did you feel, usually, during past 1 month?' It should be remembered that the time frame may vary according to the situation, which you want to address. For example, a person who had lost his spouse a year back, this time frame can be 1 year instead of 1 month (Fig. 1.2.2).

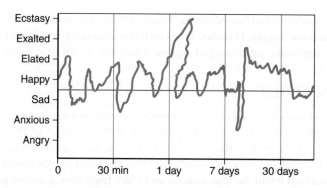

FIGURE 1.2.2

Qualitative and quantitative variations in mood over time.

After mood, you should enquire for *perceptual disturbances*. Perception is different from sensation. Right now when you are reading this line, a muffled voice of fan may be reaching your ear and auditory cortex, image of all the nearby objects are falling on your retina and reaching the visual cortex, but you may be consciously recognizing only the words printed here. What all is reaching to the cortex is sensation and what you are able to consciously acknowledge is perception. This perception is usually influenced by emotional state of brain—if you are enjoying the reading you may not be perceiving other sensations. Perceptual disturbances include illusions (altered perception of an external stimulus, eg, mistaking a rope for snake or vice versa) and hallucinations (experiences in absence of an external stimulus). In psychiatry practice, we usually encounter auditory hallucinations and visual hallucinations. They should be differentiated not only by illusions but also by imagery, also known as fantasy. Just try to imagine your house from outside or any song sung by Kishore Kumar. You can appreciate the image or the voice but these are not clear, rather they are vivid. This imagery is under voluntary control—when you think about something else, these fantasies go away; you can appreciate that they are inside your head. When you focus on the front gate of your house, surroundings start fading. When and as long as you keep imagining these fantasies, your brain gets disconnected from outside world. These qualities are not seen in hallucinations. Contrary to imagery, hallucinations are clear; one can appreciate normal perception from the sensory modality through which he/she is hallucinating (person with auditory hallucinations will be able to hear hallucinatory voices along with the environmental noises), person does not have any voluntary control over hallucinations and he/she can appreciate that they are outside his/her personal space and that they are reaching through any of the special senses to his/her brain.

Speech sample:
Doctor: Your family members reported that you keep on muttering. They also report that you do not have a habit of talking to yourself. They are noticing it for past 15 days. Do you hear some voices that other can't hear?
Patient: Yes, I do hear some voices from my neighbourhood. They talk about me all the time.
Doctor: How many people are they? Can you recognize them?
Patient: They are three. I can't recognize them.
Doctor: What happens when you try to engage yourself in some other activity to distract your attention?
Patient: No matter what do I do, I can't stop these voices.

Doctor: Are you able to appreciate other noises as well, when you hear these voices? Let's consider you are watching a movie on TV. What happens to these voices at that time?
Patient: They keep coming! They trouble me in listening and focusing on the dialogues.
Doctor: Do you think, these voices emerge inside you or they come from outside.
Patient: No doc! These voices do not belong to me. They come from outside.

Lastly, we examine for *thoughts*. We look for the flow of thought, whether he/she is able to maintain normal flow or is it restricted or there is paucity of thoughts. People with depression often have paucity of thoughts and flow is restricted; a reverse picture may be seen in anxious people. Thus, depressed persons talk slowly and use minimum words. Patients with schizophrenia or delirium may show derailment of thoughts, ie, they speak copiously, but their thoughts are not interconnected. Similarly, patients with mania may take clues from their thoughts and keep on talking for long time, switching from one subject to another, but always taking clues from the previous thought (flight of ideas) (Fig. 1.2.3).

During the thought examination, you must also try to assess the delusions, if the patient has any! This is a tricky issue and requires considerable experience to establish. When you are examining the delusions, make sure that the belief is 'not shared by other people in the community', 'false', 'firm and unshakable'. To shake the belief you must gently challenge it by presenting contradictory evidences. If despite presenting contradictory evidences, patient holds the belief, you may label it delusion.

Speech sample:
Doctor: Your mother said that you don't like your friend.
Patient: Yes doc! He was my good friend but for past 3 months he has started behaving strangely. He always makes fun of me. He is damaging my reputation.
Doctor: But your mother does not believe this. Does anybody else at your workplace believe this?
Patient: I had a talk with my other colleagues. They say that I am mistaking somewhere. He is a good guy.
Doctor: Why would he try to do this? What will he get by doing so?
Patient: He wants me out of this office because I am at a better position than him. He wants to occupy my position.

Like this you should try to assess the firmness and conviction of the belief.

With this, we complete the examination of a psychiatric patient. Always remember, dealing with psychiatric patients require skill because you are dealing with disordered emotions. A wrong move (overdoing, judgmental remarks, imparting your beliefs on patient) may disrupt the therapeutic relationship and interfere with the diagnostic and therapeutic process.

SUMMARY

- History taking is an important part as in other medical branches.
- Medical and neurological history is important because these factors may disrupt brain's functioning and produce psychiatric symptoms.
- Psychiatric examination is incomplete without medical and neurological examinations.

1. Normal Speech

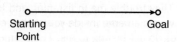

2. Circumstantial Speech
(Over-inclusive)

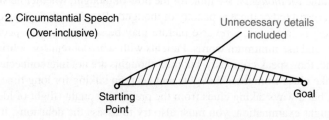

3. Tangential Speech

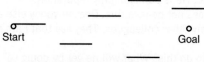

4. Derailment of Speech

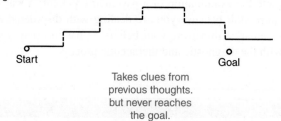

5. Flight of ideas

Start

Goal

Takes clues from
previous thoughts.
but never reaches
the goal.

FIGURE 1.2.3

Examination of the thought flow.

CLASSIFICATION OF PSYCHIATRIC DISORDERS: CHANGING CONCEPTS

1.3

Ravi Gupta

We have a number of medical disorders and many of them share one or more features with other disorders. Some of them belong to a particular system, eg, both congestive heart failure and myocarditis are cardiac disorders, Parkinson disease and Alzheimer disease are neurological disorders, and so on. Similarly, many of them have one or more symptoms in common, eg, both asthma and myocardial infarction may present with episodic breathlessness; both dementia and delirium show memory disturbances. Adding some more to the list, some disorders have shared pathophysiology, eg, ileitis and laryngitis are infectious diseases; pellagra and night blindness are nutritional disorders. So what did you see? We have classified the disorders based on the system that they affect, based on the clinical presentation and, lastly, based on aetiology. Thus, any medical disorder may be classified in different ways and each classification system depicts a particular quality.

However, as a clinical scientist, a question should come to your mind—'What is the need for classifying the medical disorders?

The answer is

1. First and foremost, classification reduces the burden of all the information that we need to remember.
2. Classification gives us an idea which system of the body we are dealing with.
3. It also tells us about the pathophysiological process and thus we can plan the treatment accordingly.
4. It guides us to the differential diagnosis.

As you have seen, all the four points mentioned above indicate the importance of classification for you as an individual. However, the scope of classification of medical disorders goes beyond individual level. Let us assume that somebody had fallen sick while on a visit to a foreign land, especially one with linguistic differences. For example, a person with major depressive disorder who is continuing the treatment from India or any other English-speaking country visits Germany or France. He experiences a relapse there and decides to consult somebody. Unfortunately, the doctor whom he consults there does not know English and because of this linguistic barrier, the physician in the foreign land will not be able to get any idea regarding the illness and its treatment until he gets an interpreter. Imagine the impact of this kind of situation on the patient who has coronary artery disease or is recovering from a stroke and experiences the same again! To deal with such situations, wise medical scientists came with a concept not only to classify all the medical disorders but also to codify them using English alphabets and Arabic numbers. Thus, 'classification and coding' helps us to communicate with each other beyond the linguistic barrier, e.g., depression is depicted as 'F-32' in International Classification of Disease-10 (ICD-10), proposed by the World Health Organization in 1992. These alphanumeric codes can be conveyed to medical persons anywhere in the world and they can search for the disease name in ICD-10. English alphabets and Arabic numerals were chosen because these are followed in most of the countries. To conclude, we can say that 'classification and coding' of medical disorders helps us to reduce the burden on memory, improves our understanding towards a disease and helps us to communicate with the medical fraternity beyond linguistic barriers.

So far, we have discussed about the utility of the classification system. In the subsequent sections, we will discuss the major classification systems that are being followed worldwide and what do they add to psychiatry practice.

CLASSIFICATION SYSTEMS

Astute medical scientists at the World Health Organization classified all the medical disorders that were known in 1992 and provided this document a name—International Classification of Diseases (ICD-10);'10' represents that this is the 10th revision of the classification system. It is periodically revised to incorporate latest information regarding the old disorders, to include disorders that have been discovered since the last revision and to remove or modify the nomenclature wherever appropriate. Similarly, the United States proposed a separate classification system known as Diagnostic and Statistical Manual (DSM) and presently we have its fifth edition (DSM-5). DSM-5 was floated in 2013, whereas ICD-10 is approximately 20 years old and currently under revision.

WHAT DO THEY ADD TO PSYCHIATRY PRACTICE?

We have already discussed in the introductory chapter that psychiatry is still evolving and that major changes have appeared after the invention of functional neuroimaging techniques. These techniques are helping us to understand the neurobiology of psychiatric disorders since the past 20 years. However, before that we knew very little about the neurobiology and hence most of the disorders were classified phenomenologically, ie, based on the similarity or proximity of symptoms. To give you some examples—all the disorders where anxiety was a major problem were clubbed under Anxiety Disorders; where mood was a major problem were clubbed under Mood Disorders, and so on. This approach was followed by ICD-10 as well as by DSM till its fourth text revision (DSM-IV-TR). But you need to understand that the phrase 'birds of a feather flock together' does not always holds true and there are fair chances that disorders with similar symptoms may have dissimilar pathology. For example, hemiplegia of upper motor neuron type may occur due to cortical injury, due to an injury to internal capsule, due to an injury in the brain stem, and so on! Similarly, anxiety may be seen during dyspnoea, during hypoglycaemia, during generalized anxiety disorder or during alcohol withdrawal or cannabis intoxication.

Medical scientists realized the shortcoming of phenomenological classification while preparing DSM-5 and classified psychiatric disorders based on neurobiological mechanisms. Thus, this system is different from ICD-10. To make the issue clearer, considering the neurobiological differences between anxiety disorders and obsessive–compulsive disorder, DSM-5 has removed it from the group of anxiety disorders and mentioned it as a separate entity.

However, DSM-5 does not remove phenomenological basis in entirety as we are still in the process of unwinding the complexities of the operational brain and have a limited knowledge regarding the neurobiology of many of the psychiatric disorder. Thus, at its best, both of these classification systems should be considered as *guidelines* that classify, name and codify various behavioural disorders.

It must be noted that symptomatology of various psychiatric disorders was similar in these two classification systems; still, they had some important differences. It had a negative impact while translating the research into clinical practice, as the symptomatology of a disorder varied between ICD-10 and DSM-5. Thus, what is schizophrenia as per the ICD-10 may be schizophreniform disorder as per DSM-5. Medical scientists have also acknowledged the problems arising out of these discrepancies and attempts are being made to bridge these gaps in the forthcoming version of the ICD, ie, ICD-11, which is expected to appear in 2017. Moreover, DSM is followed in the Unites States, whereas most of the other countries follow ICD.

Therefore, this book is based on the DSM-5 system, though we have provided comparable taxonomy from ICD-10 as well.

HOW TO USE DSM OR ICD FOR PSYCHIATRY PRACTICE?

As we have already discussed that description of psychiatric disorders is still largely phenomenological and ICD and DSM descriptions are the best be considered as *guidelines*. I have seen many people who open any of these classification systems and start matching the patient's symptoms with the symptoms mentioned in the book and arrive to a diagnosis, especially in psychiatry. However, this approach is not justified as it may lead to serious errors in diagnosis. Had this been the way to diagnose medical disorders, then anybody would have opened the textbook of any of the specialty and could have started medical practice.

It must be remembered that one needs to undergo a proper residency training programme to understand the intricacies of phenomenology of disorders and their neurobiology, according to these classification systems before starting psychiatry practices. This is because people may have different expression for a given emotion, both verbally and nonverbally; similarly, different people behaving in different manners may have one underlying emotion, eg, irritability can be a normal emotion; or it can be a sign of intermittent explosive disorder or depression or schizophrenia or mania or alcohol withdrawal, and so on. Similarly, low mood and fatigue may be seen in depression, grief, major loss, adjustment disorder, congestive heart failure, chronic inflammatory conditions and Parkinson disease to name a few. Thus, a medical background and experience in psychiatry are required to use these classification systems.

FUTURE OF CLASSIFICATION IN PSYCHIATRY

We have discussed that substantial changes have been made in the classification systems in psychiatry practice since they first appeared. This has changed them from purely phenomenological to phenomeno-neurobiological, as we see in DSM-5. In future, as more of the neurobiological underpinning will be uncovered, we can expect that psychiatric disorders will be classified purely neurobiologically, eg, those affecting primarily the prefrontal cortex, or those involving amygdala!

SUMMARY

- Classification is important so as to reduce the burden on memory and to improve the conceptual understanding.
- Two major classification systems that are being followed are ICD-10 and DSM-5.
- Classification systems code all the disorders and thus help in improving communication despite linguistic barriers.
- So far, the classification in psychiatric disorders was phenomenological; however, with the advancement of research in this field, it is becoming more and more neurobiological.

INVESTIGATIONS IN PSYCHIATRY

1.4

Ravi Gupta

Like any other medical branch, investigations are the part and parcel of psychiatry practice. We have discussed that psychiatric disorders emerge because of the changes in brain functioning and any structural change in the brain can also alter its functioning; thus, almost all neurosurgical and neurological problems have psychiatric manifestations. Diagnosis of these problems may require various investigations, like CT scan or MRI scan of the brain. Similarly, any metabolic change in the body can alter the brain functioning and can induce psychiatric symptoms. These metabolic problems are diagnosed using various investigations, like serum electrolytes, blood sugar, liver function test, kidney function test and arterial blood gas analysis to name a few. Thus, a good psychiatrist must possess optimum knowledge related to indications and interpretation of various investigations.

Structural neuroimaging (CT scan and MRI) is required in psychiatry practice, especially in the cases of headache, delirium and those with neuropsychiatric symptoms. We are purposefully omitting details of structural neuroimagings as you can read it from other textbooks of medicine and surgery.

In this chapter, we will focus on functional neuroimaging and polysomnography as most of the current research in psychiatry is using functional neuroimaging techniques and sleep complaints are an integral part of psychiatry symptomatology. At present, the use of functional neuroimaging is limited to research; however, in future, they may be used to reach to a diagnosis. Lastly, sleep disturbances are an integral part of psychiatry practice; thus, as a psychiatrist, you must know various sleep disorders and their diagnostic modalities.

In addition to the detailed discussion of these two diagnostic modalities, we will also try to highlight common diagnostic modalities that are helpful in either diagnosis or management of psychiatric disorders (Table 1.4.1).

Commonly, blood counts, liver function test, kidney function test, blood glucose concentration and electrocardiogram are advised. These investigations are important for the diagnosis and finding out the comorbidities. Considering the haematotoxic, hepatotoxic, cardiotoxic and nephrotoxic potential of some of the psychotropic agents, these investigations are ordered before starting the pharmacotherapy and during the course of pharmacotherapy. Second-generation antipsychotics alter the lipid profile and it should be monitored before the initiation of therapy and periodically during the therapy.

Table 1.4.1 Common Diagnostic Modalities Used in Psychiatry

Modality	Diagnosis	Management
Complete haemogram	Delirium, chronic fatigue syndrome, anxiety, depression	Delirium, patients on antiepileptics, mood stabilizers, clozapine
Liver function test	Delirium, alcoholic liver disease	Serum AST/ALT periodically in patients on antiepileptics, agomelattine
Serum creatinine	Delirium	Patients on lithium, before starting pregabalin and gabapentin
Lipid profile		Patients on second-generation antipsychotics, alcohol dependence
Serum CPK	Neuroleptic malignant syndrome, chronic fatigue syndrome, depression	Neuroleptic malignant syndrome
Serum iron profile	Delirium, restless legs syndrome	Restless legs syndrome
ECG	Panic disorder	Before starting quetiapine, ziprasidone, clozapine, fluvoxamine, atomoxetine
Chest X-ray	To rule out pulmonary pathology in patients with opioid withdrawal, anxiety disorder	
CAT scan brain	Headache, dementia, delirium, atypical presentation of any psychiatric disorder, catatonia, intellectual disability, specific learning disorders	
MRI brain	Headache, delirium, dementia, neuropsychiatric disorders, catatonia, atypical presentation of any psychiatric disorder, intellectual disability, specific learning disorders	

PLASMA CONCENTRATION OF DRUGS

Investigative techniques are available to measure the plasma concentrations of lithium and antiepileptics. Among these, as of now, we have evidence for the measurement of serum lithium levels during the course of management when a patient is on lithium. Measurement of plasma concentration is not routine prescribed for antiepileptics in psychiatry practice.

FUNCTIONAL NEUROIMAGING

Functional neuroimaging refers to those modalities that assess the functioning of the brain and these include functional MRI (f-MRI), positron emission tomography (PET) and single photon emission computerized tomography (SPECT). We will discuss each of these one by one.

FUNCTIONAL MRI

It detects the changes in the blood flow of the brain. This is dependent upon the notion that brain areas consume oxygen when they are activated. This oxygen is delivered through blood and thus, blood flow in a given brainarea is directly proportional to its activity. In other words, areas that are most active have higher blood flow and vice versa. In this technique, the signals from the oxygenated and deoxygenated blood are measured.

In this technique, blood flow is first recorded at rest and during a task performance by the study-subject. Areas with increased blood flow correspond to the areas that are engaged in accomplishment of a given task (Fig. 1.4.1). It is a noninvasive procedure and does not require any radiotracer, thus it is safe. It also provides good spatial and temporal resolution.

POSITRON EMISSION TOMOGRAPHY

This is another method which helps us to localize receptors in addition to the measurement of blood flow. In this method, depending upon what we intend to measure (blood flow or the receptor density), a radiolabelled tracer is injected into the body. To measure the blood flow, 5-fluorodeoxyglucose is often used. Areas with high activity have higher metabolic rate and thus, they accumulate higher amounts of

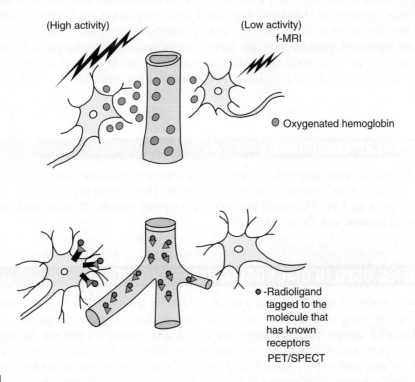

FIGURE 1.4.1

Principles of functional neuroimaging.

radiotracer than the surrounding areas, which can be measured using a nuclear imaging camera. For the receptors, the agonist or the antagonist is tagged with a radioactive material and injected into the body. This material gets attached to its respective receptor and its location and density can be measured. It has a higher spatial resolution than SPECT because in this technique, tracer emits positrons that collide with the neighbouring electrons and emit gamma photons.

SINGLE PHOTON EMISSION COMPUTERIZED TOMOGRAPHY

This technique also uses radiolabelled tracers, but unlike tracers used in PET, these tracers themselves emit gamma rays. This leads to a poor spatial resolution of the image. We can measure blood flow using ^{99m}Tc-HMPAO (hexamethylpropyline amine oxide) tracer. This tracer gets accumulated in highly active regions. The relative activity (density of gamma emissions) can be measured using gamma camera and results can be inferred.

DIAGNOSIS AND MANAGEMENT OF SUBSTANCE USE DISORDERS

People who consume addictive substances, eg, tobacco, alcohol, opioids and cannabis fall in the purview of psychiatric disorders. They often seek help for the detoxification and de-addiction; sometimes, they may present to an emergency department with intoxication. In all these conditions, it may sometimes become necessary to find out the nature of substance consumed. To identify the substance that has been consumed, dipstick tests, gas layer chromatography and other methods are available. These methods provide both qualitative (which substance was used) and quantitative (concentration of substance in blood) results, which can be used to identify the substance and to plan and monitor the therapy.

ELECTROENCEPHALOGRAPHY

Patient with delirium and epilepsy are at the interface between psychiatry and neurology. Both the specialists come across and manage these kinds of patients. Thus, a good psychiatrist must possess the basic knowledge of the EEG. He should be able to pick various epileptic disorders and must be aware of various EEG patterns seen during delirium.

MODALITIES USED IN DIAGNOSING SLEEP DISORDERS

We can use a number of modalities based on the disease in question. The simplest modality is the sleep diary or the sleep-log. This is a paper that contains the information regarding bedtime and wake-up time of a patient. This is a subjective record and patients fill this log for approximately 2 weeks (Fig. 1.4.2). Another part of this log contains the information regarding sleep hygiene and this can be used for intervention (Fig. 1.4.2). This is a relatively inexpensive method with a good reliability and gives a good estimate of subjective sleep quality, although at times information may be misleading because it depends upon the recall and subjective appreciation.

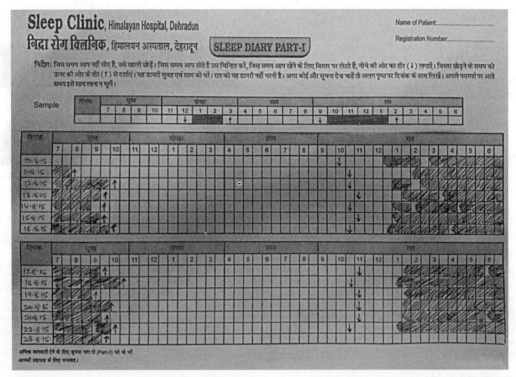

FIGURE 1.4.2

Sleep diary suggestive of delayed sleep–phase disorder.

(Source: Himalayan Hospital, Dehradun.)

To remove this recall bias, another method—actigraphy—was developed. As the name suggests, this method records the activity of a person using a watch-like instrument, which is to be worn on the nondominant wrist. It has a motion sensor that records the movements and periods of quiescence are considered as periods of sleep. These data can be downloaded using software and sleep patterns can be assessed (Fig. 1.4.3). This method provides an objective assessment of the sleep–wake period; however, it may also be misleading at times. One of the major limitations is the fact that it does not give any idea about the quality of sleep. Secondly, many patients of insomnia keep lying in bed without making significant movements and these periods of quiescence may be mistaken for sleep. On the contrary, some of the patients may have periodic movements during sleep, eg, those having restless legs syndrome, obstructive sleep apnoea to name a few and, in them periods of sleep may be mistaken for wakefulness.

Another investigation that is useful in the diagnosis of sleep-related disorders is polysomnography, also known as sleep study. This is a recording of multiple physiological parameters during sleep. The data are recorded in the software during night and the next day it is manually scored by a trained sleep-technician or sleep-physician. Depending upon the complexity, it can be of various types, as mentioned in Table 1.4.2.

For the diagnosis of sleep disorders, level I polysomnography is considered gold standard, provided that a trained scorer has scored the data manually.

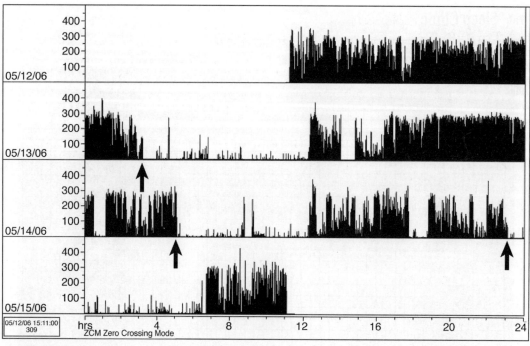

FIGURE 1.4.3

Actigraph and its data.

SUMMARY

- Psychiatry is a branch of medicine, hence investigations are required.
- Certain investigations are required for diagnosis, whereas others are required for treatment.
- Functional imaging techniques that are presently used for the research may become the diagnostics after adequate data are collected.

Table 1.4.2 Types of Polysomnography

	Level I Study	Level II Study	Level III Study	Level IV Study
Technician	Present	Absent	Absent, may be present	Absent
Place	Laboratory	Home	Home/laboratory	Home/laboratory
Channels	EEG: 6 channels Electrooculogram EMG chin and leg Airflow: thermister and pressure transducer both Respiratory movements: RIP belts chest and abdomen Oxygen saturation EKG: 2 channels Snore microphone Synchronized audio–visual recording Capnography for children	EEG: 6 channels Respiratory movement Airflow EKG Electrooculogram EMG chin and leg Oxygen saturation Snore microphone	Respiratory movement Airflow Oxygen saturation ECG	Pulse oximetry ECG
Cost effectiveness	**Most useful, can pick almost all sleep disorders**	10% patients are misclassified, may require repetition of the study in a sleep laboratory	Only for screening. *According to American Academy of Sleep Medicine unattended level III studies are not recommended to either rule in or rule out Obstructive Sleep Apnoea (OSA)*	Poor sensitivity and specificity for diagnosing and confirming OSA

INTELLECTUAL DISABILITY

2.1

Mohan Dhyani and Ravi Gupta

Intellectual disability (ID; earlier known as mental retardation) is a heterogeneous group of disorders where the hallmark is markedly reduced intellectual abilities leading to impairment in adaptive functioning. The intellectual ability or intelligence varies in a population. Thus, an individual having a lesser intelligence compared to his peer group is not considered to be intellectually disabled, unless there is some impairment in adaptive functioning.

The diagnosis is not based solely on low score in the test of intelligence quotient (IQ). Fundamentally, IQ tests are usually based on a composite score for a variety of cognitive abilities, such as mathematical calculations, language, general awareness and abstract reasoning. These abilities vary with culture, literacy and training. The IQ tests that are validated in one population (eg, in students of a metropolitan city) may not be valid in another population (eg, uneducated village-dwelling population). The performance in these tests, therefore, needs to be seen in context of other factors.

Grossly ID may be conceptualized to be composed of two groups. The first group is the population that falls in the lower range of the normal distribution curve. Here no other neuropsychiatric or genetic syndrome is evident. The intellectual functioning in this group is usually impaired in mild to moderate form. The second group comprises severe or profound ID cases and these are usually secondary to a chromosomal defect or comorbid neuropsychiatric disorders.

NOSOLOGY

The DSM-5 refers to the disorder as 'intellectual disability', whereas the ICD-10 categorized it as 'mental retardation'.

VIGNETTE

An 8-year-old boy was brought to the outpatients department with complaints of not being able to study, inability to communicate properly and age inappropriate behaviour. The parents report that the developmental milestones in the child were attained after a delay. He was able to walk only at the age of 3 years. He learned to talk in short phrases by the age of 5 years. The child was admitted in school at 6 years of age but he has not been able to learn any alphabets. He could not follow the directions of the teacher and schooling had to be discontinued. The child is only able to speak in short sentences and is not able to recognize colours. He tries to play with other children but is unable to as he does not understand the rules of the games. There is no history of seizures or any other physical deformity in the child. There is no family history of any psychiatric illness. Based on the global impairment in cognitive functioning, diagnosis of ID was made.

CLINICAL PICTURE

The signs and symptoms of ID appear from early childhood. The developmental milestones, such as head control, sitting with support, walking, babbling and talking, may be delayed. The delay may be more evident in severe and profound disability where the child takes noticeably longer period to learn to walk or talk. In milder disability, the problems are first noticed in school, where the child is slow to learn and unable to keep up with his/her peers. The child is not able to build friendship with his peers and play with them, not for the effort of trying, but because he is not able to understand the rules of the games and is not able to communicate properly.

In adults, the symptoms depend on the severity of ID. Mild ID may go unnoticed throughout life. On the other hand, severe and profound ID in adults may be confused with other psychiatric disorders, more so, if a reliable informant is not available to give developmental history. Although, ID manifests from childhood, but the disorder is not exclusive to childhood age. Any adult presenting with abnormal behaviour, where the psychotic symptoms, like delusions and hallucinations, are not clearly evident, a diagnosis of 'ID' should be ruled out.

The severity of ID was earlier categorized on the basis of IQ. But, since IQ tests are not always customized to different populations, the performance on these tests alone may not be sufficient to categorize severity. The severity of illness is based on the impairment in adaptive function in addition to the decrement in intellectual functions.

MILD ID

People with mild ID are usually able to take care of activities of daily living (ADL). Assistance is required in complex task, such as money management, legal matters and decisions regarding health care. They can be trained and may acquire vocational skills with minimal support.

MODERATE ID

People with moderate ID may be able to take care of ADL, and may achieve vocation in unskilled work and be able to work under supervision. They usually require supervision in outdoor activities like travelling and money management.

SEVERE ID

People with severe ID require constant supervision. These patients may be able to contribute to some of the ADL after training and can perform simple tasks. However, it is not possible to train such people for any vocational work.

PROFOUND ID

People with profound ID require care and assistance in almost all the activities. They are unable to perform tasks like eating and bathing. Speech development is minimal in them.

In addition, a child's general physical examination and neurological examination may also throw a light on the possible aetiology (Fig. 2.1.1).

However, in most of the patients, no specific cause may be found for the ID. ID is a heterogeneous group of disorders and clinical picture may vary a lot. Some common genetic syndromes that present with ID are shown in Table 2.1.1.

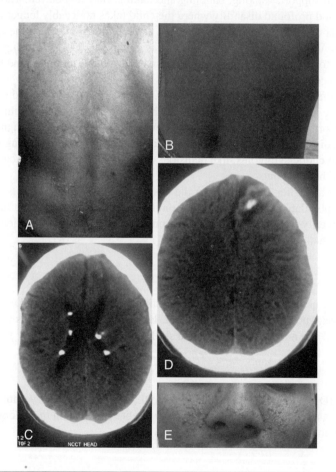

FIGURE 2.1.1

General Physical examination and investigations may throw a light on underlying aetiology. All these symptoms are seen in tuberous sclerosis. (A) Shagreen patch, (B) café-au-lait spots, (C) subependymal calcifications in the CT scan of the brain, (D) subcortical calcification in the CT scan of the brain, (E) adenoma sebaceum.

(Source: Himalayan Hospital, Dehradun.)

Table 2.1.1 Common Genetic Disorders with Intellectual Disability

Disorder	Pathology	Clinical Features
Down syndrome	Trisomy 21	Upward slanted palpebral fissures, small chin, wide nasal bridge, single crease of palm (simian crease), hypotonia, increased congenital heart disease and thyroid abnormalities Most common cause of inherited ID
Fragile X syndrome	Mutation (inactivation) of FMR1 gene at X chromosome.	Large protruding ears, long face, high arched palate, macroorchidism, hyperextensible joints, mitral valve prolapsed, strabismus Comorbid autism in 5% patients
Prader–Willi syndrome	Deletion in chromosome 15 (15q11–15q13) of paternal origin	Obesity, small hand and feet, soft, easily bruised skin, almond-shaped eyes, excessive sleeping, hyperphagia, cryptorchidism, short stature, scoliosis, Compulsive behaviour
Angelman syndrome (Happy puppet syndrome)	Deletion or inactivation in chromosome 15 (15q11–15q13) of maternal origin	Happy disposition, paroxysmal laughter, night-time waking, dysmorphic face, wide mouth, prominent mandible, microcephaly, seizure disorder common Fascinated with water and music
Cri-du-chat syndrome	Partial deletion, 5p chromosome	Infantile cat-like cry, micrognathia behavioural problems, self-injurious behaviour, hyperactivity Prone to respiratory and ear infections, congenital heart disease common with gastrointestinal abnormalities

In most of the patients of ID there may be a comorbid psychiatric disorder. Seizure disorders are more common in patients with severe and profound ID. Autistic spectrum disorders are common, especially with severe ID. Psychiatric disorders such as attention deficit hyperactivity disorder (ADHD), conduct disorder, mood disorders and schizophrenia are seen in these patients.

NEUROBIOLOGY

Neurobiology of the ID varies with the underlying aetiology. There is damage to the areas that are important for higher mental functions (birth asphyxia), or there may be a poor development of neurons, e.g., they show poor sprouting of dendrites that results in poor communication between them. In congenital storage diseases, neurons may be dysfunctional owing to storage of the substance in question.

EPIDEMIOLOGY AND RISK FACTORS

There is no reliable data on the global prevalence of ID. Studies from different countries have put the prevalence of ID in the range from less than 1–3%. The prevalence may be higher in low income countries due to the impact of under nutrition. Rates of ID are higher in boys.

DIFFERENCE BETWEEN ICD-10 AND DSM-5

DSM-5 focuses on the adaptive functioning than on the IQ score, whereas ICD-10 emphasizes on the IQ score for the diagnosis and severity assessment of ID.

DIFFERENTIAL DIAGNOSIS

NORMAL VARIATION

A poor scholastic performance of a child is not always indicative of underlying psychiatric illness. IQ tests need to be interpreted carefully, eg, a poorly motivated child may perform badly in an IQ test.

SPECIFIC LEARNING DISORDER

Before diagnosing a case of ID, make sure that the impairment is global and not specific to one cognitive ability.

CHILDHOOD DEPRESSION

The functional intelligence is reduced in mood disorders. We should not blindly depend on intelligence tests to diagnose ID. Make sure that the child is not depressed or having poor motivation for the IQ test.

ADHD

Poor score in an IQ test may be secondary to lack of attention. Rule out ADHD before making a diagnosis of ID.

DIAGNOSTIC FALLACIES

Almost all the psychiatric disorders result in some amount of intellectual dysfunction. If the IQ tests are performed on a psychotic or a very anxious patient, eg, the test scores of the same will be low. A diagnosis of intellectual disorder should only be made after a detailed psychiatric evaluation, where other psychiatric disorders have been ruled out.

We are talking about this continuously as traditionally IQ is considered a measure of intelligence, which can be misleading. IQ testing has its own limitations. It is just like solving a puzzle. If the child is not prepared and motivated for the test, he will not perform well. Role of the examiner under whom the child is performing the tests is also important. A child would not perform well in an unfriendly environment; on the other hand, an environment that is too friendly, it may also preclude the child from optimal performance. Score in the test also depends upon the interest of the child. If a child is not interested in the kind of puzzles or problems that he is presented with, he will not do well. We have to also take into account the educational status, sedation due to psychotropic medication and cultural background of the patient while interpreting the IQ test scores. Therefore, in the DSM-5, emphasis has been placed on the

ADL of the child rather than on the IQ. Impairment in the adaptive functions is necessary for diagnosis. These need to be assessed carefully keeping in mind that a critical parent may exaggerate whereas a protective parent may be downplaying the deficiencies of the child.

MANAGEMENT

Management of the ID involves a teamwork of multiple disciplines. In many cases, there may be a comorbid neurological or psychiatric disorder. The focus of the management is on training the patient and to the caregiver to *optimize the functioning of the patient* with realistic goals that are set keeping in mind the patients existing intellectual functions.

Education of the caregiver is essential to optimize the expectations. The caregivers require assistance and training to deal with the excessive burden of care. Vocational and social skills training, where feasible, help a great deal in long-term outcome. On the other hand, neglect and lack of training worsens the prognosis.

Pharmacotherapy options are not to be routinely exercised but may be used to treat the comorbid condition or for uncontrolled aggression and hostility. Treatments, both psychosocial and pharmacological, are symptom based.

COURSE AND PROGNOSIS

The outcome depends on the severity of disability. An early intervention with focused approach may result in a better functional outcome. However, the adaptation process continues lifelong and efforts to maximize the functioning should continue.

SUMMARY

- ID is a group of disorders where the hallmark is global impairment in functioning.
- An assessment of adaptive functions is more useful in categorizing the severity of the illness and not the IQ scores.
- Clinical picture varies with the comorbid conditions and underlying genetic disorder, if any.
- A multidiscipline and targeted training improves the outcome whereas neglecting the condition may worsen the outcome.

FURTHER READING

1. American Psychiatric Association. (2013). "Diagnostic and Statistical Manual of Mental Disorders." 5th edit, Author, Washington, DC.
2. Andres M., and Fred R. V. (Eds.). (2007). "Lewis' Child and Adolescent Psychiatry. A Comprehensive Textbook." 4th edit, Lippincott Williams & Wilkins; Philadelphia.
3. Rutter M., Bishop D., Pine D., Scott S., Stevenson J., Taylor E., and Thapar A. (Eds.). (2008). "Rutter's Child and Adolescent Psychiatry." 5th edit, Blackwell, Oxford, UK.
4. World Health Organization. (1992). "The ICD-10 Classification of Mental and Behavioural Disorders: Clinical Descriptions and Diagnostic Guidelines." Author, Geneva.

SPECIFIC LEARNING DISORDERS

2.2

Mohan Dhyani and Ravi Gupta

Specific learning disorders (SLD) are a group of neurodevelopmental disorders where there is a problem in learning and acquiring academic skills. In intellectual disability, the problems are global, affecting almost all the domains, but in SLD, the problems are more specifically related to academic performance.

Scholastic skills are different from cognitive functions, as they do not develop spontaneously with biological maturity. These skills are acquired by the process of learning. A lot of external factors affect learning, eg, quality of schooling, family environment (parents literate and assisting in studies or not) and each child's motivation and efforts. In addition, scholastic performance in normal population varies widely. So SLD is considered only when other factors are ruled out and it is clearly demonstrated that the child is persistently having a significant difficulty in one or more domains of learning.

NOSOLOGY

The categorization of SLD is different in ICD-10 and DSM-5. Table 2.2.1 shows the differences in categories.

VIGNETTE

An 8-year-old boy was referred to the child psychiatry clinic by his teacher with chief complaints of academic difficulty. The parents reported that the child had problems in learning almost all the subjects. He was doing well in mathematics earlier but was now having difficulty in that subject as well. There were no delays in developmental milestones. The child appeared motivated to learn; the parents were supportive and not critical. On examination, the child did not have any intellectual disability; he, however, had great difficulty in reading. He took longer time to read simple sentences and would break simple words while studying. He had no problems in verbal tests. He performed well in arithmetic questions, but if the same were put in written form he had a great difficulty in reading them out and solving them. He was diagnosed of having 'specific reading disorder'.

CLINICAL PICTURE

The symptoms of SLD are specific to the subtype of disorder. The child is apparently '*weak*' in one subject or another. He appears to be interested in studying and does not have any other symptoms of underlying psychiatric disorder.

IMPAIRMENT IN READING

There is a marked difficulty in being able to read the written text. Other aspects, which do not depend on fluent reading, may be unaffected and the child is good at oral discussion, art, geometry and mathematics. Reading is slow and strenuous with inability to read the whole word at a time. Fluency is greatly hampered. There is difficulty in differentiating similar sounding words or small-function words, like an, in, on, the and that. Spellings are also affected.

As reading is essential for learning other subjects, the performance in other subjects is also affected later on. For example, the child may perform well in mathematics, but if the questions are put in a language form, he has a difficulty in reading them out and solving them. The child may avoid tasks that involve reading.

Table 2.2.1 Comparative Nosology of Specific Learning Disorders

DSM-5	ICD-10
Specific learning disorder	Specific developmental disorders of scholastic skills
Subtypes	
With impairment in reading	Specific reading disorder
With impairment in written expression	Specific spelling disorder
With impairment in mathematics	Specific disorder of arithmetical skills

IMPAIRMENT IN WRITTEN EXPRESSION

Here the child has a difficulty in spelling the words correctly and hence there is a problem in writing. The incorrectly spelled word may be phonetically acceptable, eg, RITE for WRITE, KORET for CORRECT, or it may be phonetically unacceptable, eg, PTWR for PRETTY or TIPNR for TURNIP. There is no problem in reading, and other neurological, visual and hearing impairments are ruled out. Apart from the spellings, the child may have difficulty in grammar and punctuation. While writing, the written material may not be properly organized and may lack clarity (Fig. 2.2.1).

IMPAIRMENT IN MATHEMATICS

The problem here is mainly inability to learn arithmetic skills that are age appropriate. Solving mathematical problem includes *memorizing the arithmetic facts* and then applying these facts by *following a procedure* in order to solve the problems. The impairment could be as a result of problem with learning the numbers itself or it could be the inability to understand the *concept of problem solving*. In some children, a high level of anxiety is associated with mathematics that worsens the performance. So, impairment in mathematics could be due to problem in one or all of these areas. The clinical observation is on a child, who is unable to deal with numbers and age-appropriate arithmetic problems.

ASSESSMENT OF SLD

A diagnosis of SLD should not be made only on the reports of the caregiver. The patient's performance is tested on age-appropriate assignments. If that is not readily available in the clinic, then the patient may be asked to bring his books and his performance should be tested on that.

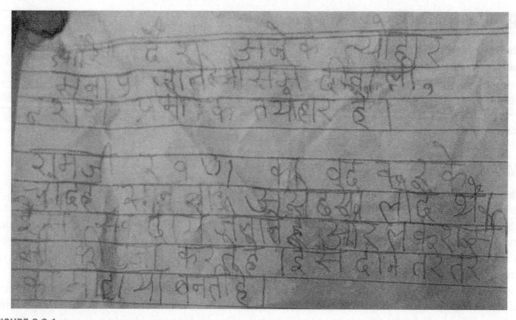

FIGURE 2.2.1

Mistakes in Hindi spellings in a child with SLD.

(Source: Himalayan Hospital, Dehradun.)

NEUROBIOLOGY

Neurobiologically, SLD involve different areas. In the mathematics disorder, primary problem has been found in right intraparietal sulcus, ventro-occipital temporal cortex and fusiform gyrus. These areas get activated during the numerical tasks. Moreover, we need prefrontal areas, eg, dorsolateral prefrontal cortex to keep the numbers in the working memory while manipulating them. Similarly, anterior cingulate cortex is important for the conflict and error monitoring that is utilized during manipulation. Decreased activity in these areas has been found in children with mathematics disorder. Left temporo-parietal cortex is involved in understanding and manipulating the language with the mathematical problems and its activity is also aberrant in these cases. Thus, in these cases right-sided dorsal fronto-parietal circuit is involved.

Similarly, for reading disorder, left side of the brain is primarily involved. It has been found that left-sided ventral-occipital cortex, fusiform gyrus, temporo-parietal cortex and inferior frontal gyrus are dysfunctional in reading disorder. These are the areas that are important for recognizing the letter, binding them into a word and to understand it. Contrary to mathematics disorder, in these cases left-sided ventral fronto-temporo-parietal circuit is involved.

Because of this neurobiological difference between two disorders, patients with combined mathematics and reading disorder are able to do the elementary calculations but not the word-based mathematical problems.

EPIDEMIOLOGY AND RISK FACTORS

The prevalence in western studies shows 5–15% prevalence among children. Among adults, the prevalence could be around 4%.

DIFFERENCE BETWEEN ICD-10 AND DSM-5

DSM-5 emphasizes that the academic difficulty persists for at least 6 months, despite the child being provided the help to overcome them. On the other hand, ICD-10 relies more on quantitative criteria and mentions that the child's score in tests for reading or comprehension or spelling or arithmetic should be 2 standard deviations below the score that is normal for that population, culture and child's age.

DIFFERENTIAL DIAGNOSIS

NORMAL VARIATION IN SCHOLASTIC PERFORMANCE

There is a wide variation in the scholastic performance of an individual. The performance depends on many extraneous factors, as we have already discussed. Poor performance in one subject does not necessarily means a diagnosis of SLD.

INTELLECTUAL DISABILITY

Although SLD can be diagnosed even in presence of intellectual disability, it needs to be ascertained that the difficulty in scholastic performance is not attributable to it.

Hearing and visual impairments should be ruled out before diagnosing SLD as should neurological disorders that may impair proper vocalization or that affect the motor skills involved in writing.

DIAGNOSTIC FALLACIES

Harsh teaching methods and parental pressure or expectation may affect academic performance. Overtly protective or critical parents may minimize or exaggerate the child's performance.

MANAGEMENT

There are no approved pharmacological interventions as of now.

Primary prevention involves giving high quality education to all students. Secondary prevention is in the form of a targeted and scientific intervention given to those who are not making academic progress, even with quality education. Tertiary prevention is individual, and special education services with educators are given to those who fail these intervention efforts.

The Central Board of Secondary Education (CBSE) of India gives concessions to students with SLD. It includes giving 15 min extra time, exemption from studying second language, allowing the use of calculator for mathematic impairment and other exemptions. (*An exhaustive list is beyond the scope of this book, readers may contact CBSE for details.*)

COURSE AND PROGNOSIS

These disorders often run a chronic course, unless adequately managed.

SUMMARY

- SLD are neurodevelopmental disorders where the scholastic performance of the child is affected.
- Poor performance in one subject does not always means presence of SLD.
- Early differentiation from intellectual disability and targeted intervention are essential.
- Outcome is good with an early intervention.

FURTHER READING

1. American Psychiatric Association. (2013). "Diagnostic and Statistical Manual of Mental Disorders." 5th edit, Author, Washington, DC.
2. Ashkenazi S., Black J. M., Abrams D. A., Hoeft F., and Menon V. (2013). Neurobiological Underpinnings of Math and Reading Learning Disabilities, *Journal of Learning Disabilities*, 46(6):549–569.
3. Kamala R. (2014). Specific Learning Disabilities in India: Rights, Issues and Challenges, *Indian Journal of Applied Research*, 4:604–605.
4. World Health Organization. (1992). "The ICD-10 Classification of Mental and Behavioural Disorders: Clinical Descriptions and Diagnostic Guidelines." Author, Geneva.

ATTENTION DEFICIT AND HYPERACTIVITY DISORDER

2.3

Mohan Dhyani and Ravi Gupta

Attention deficit and hyperactive disorder (ADHD) is a neurodevelopmental disorder with key features of overactivity/hyperactivity, inattention and impulsivity. The syndrome is also referred to as 'hyperkinetic disorder' or 'attention deficit disorder'. It is the most common childhood behavioural disorder.

When compared to adults, children are joyful, enthusiastic and energetic. It is important to differentiate this normal behaviour of a child from a behavioural disorder. The diagnosis of ADHD is considered only if the core symptoms are persistent, present in more than one setting and are causing impairment.

NOSOLOGY

In DSM-5, this disorder is termed as 'attention deficit hyperactivity disorder', whereas in ICD-10 it is mentioned as hyperkinetic disorder.

VIGNETTE

A 6-year-old boy was brought by his parents with complaints of difficulty in scholastic performance and not listening. The child is always on the move, running around and climbing on things and does not listen when called. There have been complains from school that the child does not remain seated even during a class and disturbs other children during playtime. The parents report that the academic performance of the child is affected because of careless mistakes and lack of persistence at tasks. He copies incorrectly or incompletely from the board. While studying, he gets distracted very easily and has difficulty focusing on the task in hand. The child dislikes tasks like solving puzzles or playing scrabble. Upon assessment, the child was diagnosed with ADHD.

CLINICAL PICTURE

The clinical picture of a patient varies according to age and severity of symptoms. Younger patients present with predominant hyperactivity and impulsivity, whereas the patients where inattention is predominant usually present at a later stage with difficulties in academic performance. Diagnosis of ADHD should be made only when core symptoms are present (Table 2.3.1).

The symptoms of hyperactivity are evident as a child is reported to be always on the move. The parents often describe their child as being 'driven by motor'. The child has difficulty in remaining seated at one place and when seated, is always squirming or fidgeting. The child often runs or climbs on at inappropriate situations. Adolescents may not move about that much but report inner restlessness and urge to move about. The child has difficulty in playing quietly; he talks excessively. The child is impulsive and often intrudes in other peoples' conversation or activities. He lacks the patience to wait for his turn and often blurts out answers even before the question is completed.

Table 2.3.1 Core Symptoms ADHD	
Inattention	Inability to sustain the attention on a given task, resulting in the lack of persistence and frequent change of activities
Hyperactivity or overactivity	Excessive movements for the appropriate age
Impulsivity	Acting without thinking about the consequences

In the clinic, patients with severe symptoms may be restless while waiting; child may impulsively start fidgeting with the stationary on the doctor's table or get up from their place and start moving about during the interview. Inattention is manifested as inability to focus on tasks or playful activities and a lack of persistence in these tasks. There are lots of careless mistakes by the child in the school and at home. There are problems in following the instructions and in organizing tasks and activities. The child usually dislikes activities that require sustained attention; his attention is very easily distracted by external stimulus. The child is forgetful in daily activities and often keeps on losing things, like pencils, books and lunch box.

These features should be present in more than one setting, ie, at home and in school.

NEUROBIOLOGY

Symptoms of ADHD arise due to dysfunction in the prefrontal cortex. Decreased activation of dorsolateral prefrontal cortex is responsible for deficiency in concentration. Decreased activity in the dorsal anterior cingulate gyrus underlies inability to selectively focus on a given stimulus. Thus, attention in ADHD patients keeps wandering and they are distractible. Hypofunctional orbitofrontal cortex is responsible for the impulsivity and supplementary motor area is related to the motor hyperactivity in ADHD.

This dysfunction is caused by abnormality in the dopaminergic and noradrenergic neurotransmission, since these neurotransmitters modulate the activity of the prefrontal cortex. Noradrenaline is important for recognizing the incoming stimulus (attention) and recruitment of prefrontal cortical networks, whereas dopamine prevents other less-important stimulus from reaching the prefrontal cortex (noise reduction). Thus, their optimal activity is required for the normal functioning. When the activity of these systems is too low, only a small number of signals reach the prefrontal cortex, that too with improper filtering (too much of noise). This state gives rise to the symptoms of ADHD, depending upon the cortical area where it is occurring, as stated above (Fig. 2.3.1).

EPIDEMIOLOGY AND RISK FACTORS

Attention deficit and hyperactive disorder is more predominant in boys than in girls. There is a correlation between the increasing age of the father and the incidence of ADHD in the child as well.

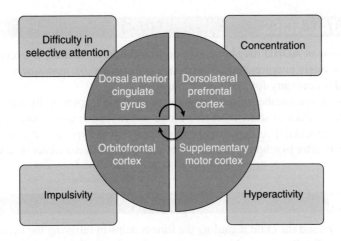

FIGURE 2.3.1

Different areas of the brain that are responsible for the symptoms of ADHD.

DIFFERENCE BETWEEN ICD-10 AND DSM-5

Description of symptoms in ICD-10 differs from DSM-5 to some extent. This is depicted in Table 2.3.2.

DIFFERENTIAL DIAGNOSIS

Poor scholastic performance may be secondary to intellectual disability, which may be misinterpreted as inattention. Similarly the scholastic performance seen in specific learning disorder (SLD) may appear as ADHD, especially if the child loses motivation and gets frustrated with the problem of SLD.

Oppositional defiant disorder (ODD) needs to be ruled out as the resistance to the demands of teachers and parents may manifest as symptoms of inattention. It should also be noted that ODD and ADHD are comorbid in many cases and presence of one should prompt the clinician to look for the other illness.

Table 2.3.2 Comparison of ICD-10 and DSM 5 Criteria[a]

DSM-5	ICD-10
Either '*inattention*' or '*hyperactivity along with impulsivity*' should be present	All three—*overactivity, inattention* and *impulsivity*— should be present
Can be diagnosed with comorbid autistic spectrum disorder	'Pervasive developmental disorder' (autistic spectrum disorder) should be ruled out
Several symptoms should be present before the age of 12 years	The symptoms should be present before 7 years of age

[a]Although the guidelines may differ, it would be prudent to focus on the concept of illness where it is described as a neurodevelopmental disorder that starts at an early age with the core symptoms described in Table 2.3.1.

DIAGNOSTIC FALLACIES

One or two symptoms of ADHD may be seen in normal children. Anxious or overenthusiastic parents and teachers may wrongly interpret normal variations as disorders. An assessment by a trained mental–health professional is necessary for a definitive diagnosis.

Inattention is seen in a number of neurocognitive disorders. Hyperactivity may be a manifestation of restlessness seen in anxious state. Increased motor activity, such as stereotypical movements seen in some neurodevelopmental disorders, may be misinterpreted as hyperactivity. A worsening of symptoms or hyperactivity after psychotropic medication could be akathasia rather than worsening illness.

MANAGEMENT

Educating the parents and the child regarding the illness helps in relieving the irritation of the parents and the guilt of the child. Behaviour therapy, with the aim of reducing the reinforcing factors and promoting adaptive behaviour, is beneficial.

Pharmacotherapy is required in children where there is significant impairment. Methylphenidate (5–10 mg/day) and atomoxetine (10–27 mg/day) have been found effective in many trials. The medication should be prescribed by trained personnel. Other medications found useful are clonidine, modafinil and imipramine have also been used with successful results in ADHD.

COURSE AND PROGNOSIS

The symptoms of ADHD usually decrease with age. Most of the patients do not have diagnosable ADHD in adulthood. However, ADHD may persist into adulthood where the symptoms of impulsivity and inattention are predominant.

SUMMARY

- ADHD is the most common behavioural disorder seen in the child and adolescent population.
- Some symptoms of inattention and hyperactivity are usual in children.
- Effective medication is available to manage the symptoms of ADHD.

FURTHER READING

1. American Psychiatric Association. (2013). "Diagnostic and Statistical Manual of Mental Disorders." 5th edit, Author, Washington, DC.
2. Stahl S. M. (2013). "Stahl's Essential Psychopharmacology." 4th edit, Cambridge University press, New Delhi, India.
3. World Health Organization. (1992). "The ICD-10 Classification of Mental and Behavioural Disorders: Clinical Descriptions and Diagnostic Guidelines." Author, Geneva.

DISRUPTIVE, IMPULSE CONTROL AND CONDUCT DISORDERS

2.4

Ravi Gupta

This group includes the disorders in which the patients have problems in controlling their emotions and behaviours. In other words, they do not have control over what they feel, often have emotions that represent the negative end of the spectrum and are not able to examine the validity of their emotions. In response to these emotions, their acts (behaviour) are often damaging to others or against the social norms. Thus, these people may be engaged in violating the rights of others.

We see two major disorders in this category—first, where primary problem is poorly controlled emotions, ie, intermittent explosive disorder, pyromania and kleptomania, and second, where primary problem is disruptive behaviour, ie, oppositional defiant disorder (ODD) and conduct disorder. Problems with controlling emotions are more common among adults; however, they are included here because of shared neurobiology.

NOSOLOGY

DSM-5 and ICD-10 have different nomenclature for these disorders, as seen in Table 2.4.1.

Table 2.4.1 Comparative Nosology of Disruptive, Impulse Control and Conduct Disorders

S. No.	DSM-5	ICD-10
1.	Oppositional defiant disorder	Oppositional defiant disorder
2.	Conduct disorder	Conduct disorder
3.	Intermittent explosive disorder	–
4.	Pyromania	Pathological fire setting
5.	Kleptomania	Pathological stealing

VIGNETTES

A 14-year-old boy was brought by the parents with complaints of behaviour that does not fit with the social norms. He has been reported to be abusive to the fellows in class and the neighbours for the last 3 years. He was indulged in physical fights mostly with the boys of same age and sometimes with elderly boys. He has been found hitting the animals without any reason. On a few occasions, he was caught stealing money from his home by his mother. On each of these occasions, he could not provide any specific reason for these acts. He is poor in studies and teachers reported missing school frequently, without informing the parents. The teachers and family members do not overrule the possibility of him being a member of a gang of similar natured adolescents, although he has never shoved his shoulder with the legal system. His mental status examination revealed that he could easily become angry, appears resentful and has no remorse over his acts. Based on the history and examination, diagnosis of conduct disorder was made.

A 26-years-old female came with her husband, as both of them were having frequent altercations for past 6 months. They have been married for 3 years and the husband noticed a change in her behaviour during this period. She often becomes irritable on trivial issues and starts yelling and damaging household articles. This episode would last for approximately half an hour and after that she feels guilty for her behavior. She says that she does not want to react in this manner and would like to change it. She expends that during the episode she has a feeling as if another person is driving her according to his wishes but she does not want to lose her control over the situation. In these circumstances, she develops extreme anger that is out of her control and associated with behavioural problems. However, between the episodes, her behaviour is completely normal. On examination, she was found to be distressed over her acts and wanted a diagnosis and treatment of the problem. Based on the history and examination, diagnosis of intermittent explosive disorder was made.

CLINICAL PICTURE

DISORDERS PRIMARILY MANIFESTED AS DISRUPTIVE BEHAVIOURS

These disorders manifest primarily as behaviours that are disruptive to the social structure and social norms. Symptoms of ODD develop during preschool years and rarely persist beyond adolescence. These can be divided into three major categories—irritability, argumentativeness and malevolent behaviour. These children often get angry on trivial issues and appear 'touchy'. When asked to do something, they often defy the authority of parents, elders and teachers. They often irritate them intentionally and then blame others for their behaviour. They are vindictive. These symptoms must last for at least 6 months before we make the diagnosis.

On the other hand, adolescents with conduct disorder have symptoms that can largely be clustered into four groups—aggression, theft, destruction of property and violation of rules. The symptoms usually start during adolescence and most of the adolescents have history of ODD during childhood. These symptoms must be present for 12 months for making the diagnosis, as disruptive behaviours may be normal emotional reactions at times. Many of the patients of conduct disorder ultimately develop antisocial personality disorder. Thus, ODD, conduct disorder and antisocial personality disorder lie on a continuum. Symptoms must interfere with personal, social and occupational functioning.

DISORDERS PRIMARILY MANIFESTED AS LOSS OF EMOTIONAL CONTROL

Intermittent explosive disorder can be diagnosed after the chronological age of 6 years. These patients often react excessively to a trivial stimulation and most of the time aggression is verbal, such as shouting, yelling and screaming at others or heated arguments that are clearly out of proportion of the context. Sometimes, physical aggression is seen and these people may damage the items that are present at the scene. However, once the anger is over, they feel distressed about it and often repent. Afterwards, they report that they were not able to control their emotions.

Kleptomania persons often steal the items without the need and often these items do not have any monetary value. They feel a 'tension' or compulsion before doing the act that is relieved after committing the act.

Pyromania may be diagnosed if the person has an impulse to set-up a fire and has tension before doing so. Fulfilment of the act provides them a sense of pleasure. The fire is setup deliberately and they have a fascination towards committing the act, often described as a curiosity—'What would happen when this object gets burnt?' However, these acts are not done for taking a revenge or for monetary benefit or as a part of criminal activity and not to express anger. Symptoms must interfere with personal, social and occupational functioning.

NEUROBIOLOGY

DISORDERS PRIMARILY MANIFESTED AS DISRUPTIVE BEHAVIOURS

These disorders are being regulated by a complex neurocircuitry that controls emotions, empathy and learning. Normally, we are able to appreciate other person's emotions and usually try to engage in those behaviours that make others happy. In these situations, amygdala functions normally and we feel a reward at the higher level, ie, ventromedial prefrontal cortex (vmPFC). In situations where the other person shows negative emotions, eg, scolding, anger and shouting (distress cues), the amygdala sends signals to the brain-stem nuclei to make us more alert and to recruit sympathetic system that has peripheral, as well as cortical effects. During this time, negativity of emotions may be appreciated at the cortical level (vmPFC).

Another part of the brain, anterior insular cortex, tells us about the emotional valence of the objects and situations. In other words, it decides what we feel. We feel both positive and negative emotions when we see the pictures with positive and negative emotions, respectively, and thus we are able to empathize emotionally. Similar to the given example of pictures for emotional empathy, while communicating we try to guess what the other person is thinking and thus try to empathize cognitively (at the level of thoughts). For cognitive empathy, we require normal functioning of vmPFC, temporo-parietal junction, temporal pole and posterior cingulate cortex. Both emotional and cognitive empathy are important for normal socialization so that we respond to different situations appropriately (Fig. 2.4.1).

Whenever we go through any emotional situation, we act in a certain fashion. If we get expected results, we repeat the same behaviour and if we get negative outcome, we try to behave in a different manner should the same situation arise in future. Dorsolateral prefrontal cortex (dlPFC) and anterior

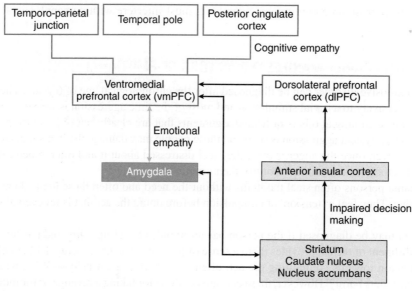

FIGURE 2.4.1

Neurobiology of disruptive disorders.

insula inhibits the response in situations of negative outcome (punishment). In other words, once we face punishment in a certain situation by some of our act (stimulus), these regions prohibit us to do the same act (stimulus) so as to prevent us from punishment (outcome).

Thus, we keep trying different strategies till we get a perfect answer that increases the chances of having positive outcome in a similar situation. Thus, we are able to associate the outcome (reward or punishment) with the stimulus (how we behave). In other words, by analysing the outcome of our action, we learn. We learn how to react to similar situation in future. This is done by the actions of amygdala, striatum (that includes caudate and nucleus accumbens) and vmPFC. This is also important for socialization and keeping the situations/relationships stable.

People with ODD or conduct disorder have normal cognitive empathy but lack the emotional empathy. In other words, they are not able to understand what the other person is feeling. Thus, they may appear fearless in dangerous situations and when they inflict the pain to anybody, they are not able to appreciate what the other person is feeling. In the brain, they show reduced functioning of amygdala, vmPFC and anterior insula. Similarly, they show dysfunctions in the other areas that are important for decision making (striatum, amygdala and vmPFC) and those that proscribe the negative outcome (dlPFC and anterior insula).

DISORDERS PRIMARILY MANIFESTED AS LOSS OF EMOTIONAL CONTROL

Our understanding of the neurobiology of these disorders is limited. However, available evidence suggests that they represent a dysfunction in amygdala–vmPFC circuitry along with the dysfunctional anterior cingulate cortex. Dopamine and serotonin neurotransmissions have been implicated in the impulsivity and aggression. Thus, these disorders share neurobiology with ODD, conduct disorders and addiction.

EPIDEMIOLOGY AND RISK FACTORS

Oppositional defiant disorder is reported in approximately 3% children with male predominance. One-year population prevalence of conduct disorder is around 4% in the United States. Prevalence is higher among males and increases till adolescence. Intermittent explosive disorder is more common in younger population as compared to older. Prevalence of pyromania and kleptomania is not known.

DIFFERENCE BETWEEN ICD-10 AND DSM-5

Largely, the criteria between two classification systems are similar.

DIFFERENTIAL DIAGNOSIS

Oppositional defiant disorder should be differentiated from conduct disorder, attention deficit hyperactivity disorder (ADHD), disruptive mood dysregulation disorder (DMDD) and intermittent explosive disorder. Children with DMDD have more frequent anger spells; these outbursts are more severe and often run a chronic course. In addition, these anger spells are superimposed upon a chronically low mood in DMDD. Unlike patients with intermittent explosive disorder, patients with oppositional defiant disorder do not show any remorse. Children with ADHD do not pay attention to the instructions rather than defying it.

Conduct disorder should be differentiated from ADHD, depressive disorder, bipolar disorder and emotional reactions due to adjustment disorder. Children and adolescent with ADHD may unknowingly engage in destructive activities because of hyperactivity. However, they do not get the pleasure out of these activities. Persons with depressive disorder are often irritable and complain of sadness of mood. Patients with bipolar disorder are seldom destructive unless they have persecutory delusions. Besides, in both of these disorders, primary problem is with mood rather than with conduct. Adolescents undergo a lot of physical and hormonal transformation that may make their brain vulnerable to act in amusing manners at times. In the situation of emotional burden, they may be engaged in acts that may be similar to those seen in conduct disorder. Before making the diagnosis of conduct disorder, one should rule out emotional reactions in adolescents.

Intermittent explosive disorder should be differentiated from DMDD, antisocial personality disorder, borderline personality disorder, substance intoxication and withdrawal and other disorders described in this chapter. In DMDD, mood is chronically low and illness starts below the age of 10 years. Antisocial personality disorder and borderline personality disorder are characterized by less intense aggression as compared to intermittent explosive disorder. A history of recent consumption of substances of abuse in large amount and that of quitting a substance after chronic use differentiates the intermittent explosive disorder from intoxication and withdrawal, respectively.

Pyromania should be differentiated from fire-setting in response to any delusion or hallucinations or epilepsy. Kleptomania should be differentiated from intentional theft or one that happens in response to delusions and hallucinations. Many a times, people with intentional stealing may malinger kleptomania to avoid criminal charges.

DIAGNOSTIC FALLACIES

1. Child who is not able to follow the commands in school because of specific learning disorder or not able to adjust in social circumstances because of autistic spectrum disorder may show temper tantrums and may be mistaken for ODD.
2. Patients with brain injury, intellectual disability and neurocognitive disorders may have anger outburst, which may be mistaken for intermittent explosive disorder.
3. Patients may set fire intentionally for the profit, to hide any criminal evidences, to take revenge or out of curiosity in the case of children. This should not be mistaken for pyromania.

MANAGEMENT

For ODD and conduct disorder, behaviour therapies are the mainstay of treatment. A number of therapies are available, eg, anger control training, group assertiveness training, incredible years, multidimensional treatment, foster care and multisystem therapy.

To control the impulsivity and aggression, antiepileptic drugs, eg, carbamazepine (10–15 mg/kg of body weight) or valproate (15–25 mg/kg of body weight), may be given. Antidepressants, particularly selective serotonin reuptake inhibitors (SSRI), also have a role in controlling impulsivity. Any of the SSRIs, eg, fluoxetine (20–80 mg/day), sertraline (50–200 mg/day), paroxetine (12.5–37.5 mg/day), may be chosen depending upon side effect profile. In selected cases, antipsychotics, eg, risperidone (2–12 mg/day) or quitiapine (50–300 mg/day), may be given.

COURSE AND PROGNOSIS

Oppositional defiant disorder often precedes conduct disorder. Children with ODD are predisposed to develop impulse control disorders. The course of conduct disorder is variable. Impulse control disorders have both episodic and persistent chronic course.

SUMMARY

- Disruptive and impulse control disorders have shared pathophysiology.
- Impulse control disorders are seen in adolescents and adults as well.
- ODD, conduct disorder and antisocial personality disorder lie on a continuum.
- Antiepileptic medications and SSRIs are important in management of aggression and impulsivity.
- These disorders must be differentiated from bipolar disorder and schizophrenia spectrum disorders.

FURTHER READING

1. American Psychiatric Association. (2013). "Diagnostic and Statistical Manual of Mental Disorders." 5th edit, Author, Washington, DC.
2. Blair R. J. (2013). The Neurobiology of Psychopathic Traits in Youths. *Nature Reviews Neuroscience*, 14:786–799.
3. Eyberg S. M., Nelson M. M., and Boggs S. R. (2008). Evidence-Based Psychosocial Treatments for Children and Adolescents With Disruptive Behavior. *Journal of Clinical Child & Adolescent Psychology*, 37:215–237.
4. World Health Organization. (1992). "The ICD-10 Classification of Mental and Behavioural Disorders: Clinical Descriptions and Diagnostic Guidelines." Author, Geneva.

FEEDING AND ELIMINATION DISORDERS

2.5

Ravi Gupta

Feeding and elimination disorders are the conditions that deal with abnormality in feeding and excretion of the child. Feeding disorders include ingestion of nonedible substances or eating behaviour that results in impairment in physical health. Elimination disorders include excretion during abnormal conditions, eg, during sleep.

NOSOLOGY

There is some difference in nomenclature between DSM-5 and ICD-10. It is depicted in Table 2.5.1.

VIGNETTE

A 10-year-old boy was brought by the family members because he was not gaining proper weight. The mother reported that the boy is too selective about the food and does not eat anything except for fried potato and, occasionally, some of the fruits. The boy appeared thin built and his weight and height were below normal for his age and gender. His mother reported that he does not eat other food simply because he does not like the smell of the vegetables and pulses. She also complained that the boy urinates during sleep and never achieved bladder control. Because of these reasons, the family is not able to stay away from home during the night and they have not gone on vacations for the past 6 years. He was diagnosed with avoidant/restrictive food intake disorder along with enuresis.

Table 2.5.1 Comparative Nosology of Feeding and Elimination Disorders	
DSM-5	**ICD-10**
Feeding disorders	
Pica	Pica of infancy and childhood
Rumination disorder	Feeding disorder of infancy and childhood
Avoidant/restrictive food intake disorder	–
Elimination disorders	
Enuresis	Nonorganic enuresis
Encopresis	Nonorganic encopresis

CLINICAL PICTURE

FEEDING DISORDERS

Pica presents with the complaints of eating nonedible substances, eg, chalk, soil and paper. Since such actions are common among infants and some toddlers, hence, this disorder is diagnosed when this practice is seen after appropriate development of the child. This disorder may also be seen among adults.

Rumination disorder presents with regurgitation of food after eating it. Patient may chew or reswallow or spit the regurgitated food material. However, it is important to rule out gastrointestinal problems before diagnosing rumination disorder.

Avoidant/restrictive food intake disorder is diagnosed when a person has selective feeding habits and avoids certain food because of their smell or the appearance. This condition may lead to weight loss or failure to thrive and/or nutritional deficiency. This must be considered that the food habits are learned and governed by the culture. Thus, any person who has not learnt to have a particular type of food will try to avoid it in certain conditions. In those conditions, this disorder should not be diagnosed. These patients sometimes need enteral feeding through nasogastric tube to meet the nutritional demands.

ELIMINATION DISORDERS

Enuresis is the most common illness, among all conditions described in this chapter. Parents usually present with the complaints that the child wets his pants. The problem may be limited to sleep (nocturnal) or may be seen during awakened state (diurnal). Nocturnal enuresis can be seen whenever the child is sleeping, either during the day or at night. Many a times, the child may wake up and find himself wet; however, at other times he comes to know about it only after he is made to wake up. However, as we have discussed, sleep is not important for the diagnosis and it may be seen during awakened state as well (diurnal enuresis). The voiding may be voluntary but is usually unintentional.

Encopresis presents with repeated passage of stool at inappropriate places. Most of the time it is involuntary, but sometimes it may be intentional. It may be associated with constipation and overflow incontinence. Stool form may vary from liquid to solid. If it is associated with constipation, symptoms usually resolve with the treatment of constipation.

A comparison of the symptomatology is depicted in Table 2.5.2.

NEUROBIOLOGY

Neurobiological underpinnings of these disorders are not well understood at present. However, certain other medical conditions may give rise to symptoms of these disorders, as mentioned in the 'Clinical Picture' and 'Differential Diagnosis'.

EPIDEMIOLOGY AND RISK FACTORS

Prevalence of feeding disorders is unknown. *Pica* usually starts during childhood, although it is not uncommon during adulthood. It is usually seen with intellectual disability. *Rumination disorder* also can

Table 2.5.2 Comparison of Clinical Picture of different Disorders

	Feeding Disorders			Elimination Disorders	
Pica	**Rumination Disorder**	**Avoidant/ Restrictive Food Intake Disorder**		**Enuresis**	**Encopresis**
Eating of nonfood substances	Repeated regurgitation of food	Lack of interest in eating food or avoidance of certain types of food or avoidance of food due to any aversive consequences		Repeated voiding in cloths or in bed. It may be intentional or involuntary	Repeated defecation at inappropriate places, eg, floor or clothes
Eating behaviour out of cultural food practices	Symptoms not explained by GERD, pyloric stenosis or other feeding and eating disorders	Associated with weight loss or nutritional deficiency or dependent on enteral feeding for meeting nutritional requirements or interference with social functioning		Child must be at least 5 years old (chronological/ mental age)	Chronological and mental age must be at least 4 years
Symptoms must last for at least 1 month	Symptoms must last for at least 1 month	–		At least twice a week for a minimum of 3 months	At least once a month for a minimum of 3 months

occur at any age. It may be a relapsing–remitting condition or it may run a chronic course. *Avoidant/ restrictive food intake disorder* may also arise at any age and may run a chronic course.

Prevalence of enuresis decreases with age–around 10% below 5 years to 1% in 15 years or older. Encopresis has a prevalence of around 1% with male predominance.

DIFFERENCE BETWEEN ICD-10 AND DSM-5

ICD-10 and DSM-5 differs in the description of symptomatology. This is depicted in Table 2.5.3.

DIFFERENTIAL DIAGNOSIS

All feeding disorders must be differentiated from one another and from eating disorders.

Rumination disorder must be differentiated from gastroesophageal reflux disorder, pyloric stenosis, gastroparesis and Sandifer syndrome.

Avoidant/restrictive food intake disorder should be differentiated from food allergies, intolerance to certain foods, neurological disorders affecting apparatus of swallowing, restricted interests seen in autistic spectrum disorder and social anxiety disorder (fear of eating in public).

Table 2.5.3 Difference in ICD-10 from DSM-5

Pica	Rumination Disorder	Avoidant/ Restrictive Food Intake Disorder	Enuresis	Encopresis
Symptoms must be seen at least twice a week for a minimum of 1 month Chronological and mental age must be at least 2 years		–	At least twice a week under 7 years of age and at least once a week after 7 years of age	Duration of disorder is at least 6 months

Enuresis must be differentiated from neurogenic bladder, diabetes mellitus, diabetes insipidus and use of some medications, eg, antipsychotics or diuretics. It is also seen in children with obstructive sleep apnoea.

Encopresis must be differentiated from spina bifida, anal stenosis and chronic diarrhoea.

DIAGNOSTIC FALLACIES

Some pregnant women may develop habit of eating nonfood substances (especially chalk), but in those cases it should be diagnosed only if it poses a medical threat.

MANAGEMENT

Feeding disorders are often managed by improving the interaction between the mother and the child. For rumination disorder, aversive therapy, eg, instilling the lemon juice in the child's mouth after rumination may help. Gastrokinetics (eg, domperidone) have been found useful in this disorder.

For enuresis, best method is the use of pad with the alarm that rings when the child wets the bed. In the evening, liquids may be restricted; anticholinergic antidepressants (eg, imipramine 10 mg/day) may be used for increasing the tone of bladder sphincter.

COURSE AND PROGNOSIS

Pica may follow a chronic course. *Rumination disorder* may be a relapsing–remitting condition or it may run a chronic course. *Avoidant/restrictive food intake disorder* may run a chronic course. *Enuresis* runs a chronic course if its symptoms persist during adolescence. *Encopresis* may be a persistent condition with occasional exacerbations.

SUMMARY

- Feeding disorders may present with medical emergencies.
- Feeding disorders may run a chronic course.
- Enuresis is associated with significant limitation in social activities.
- Other medical disorders must be excluded before diagnosing feeding and elimination disorders.

FURTHER READING

1. American Psychiatric Association. (2013). "Diagnostic and Statistical Manual of Mental Disorders." 5th edit, Author, Washington, DC.
2. World Health Organization. (1992). "The ICD-10 Classification of Mental and Behavioural Disorders: Clinical Descriptions and Diagnostic Guidelines." Author, Geneva.

AUTISTIC SPECTRUM DISORDER

2.6

Mohan Dhyani and Ravi Gupta

Autism spectrum disorders (ASD) are a group of disorders that are evident in early childhood and manifest through the lifetime. It is a heterogeneous group of disorders, earlier known as 'pervasive developmental disorders'. The hallmark of these disorders is qualitative impairment in social interactions, impaired communication and a restrictive pattern of interests and activities.

For the proper growth of a child, forming a relationship with the caregiver is necessary. Normal child is interested in the environment around it and explores it enthusiastically. From the early stages, a child has innate ability to identify other people around him and to attract their attention and communicate with them. In ASD, this ability seems to be impaired. The child appears to be reluctant to make social relations. In addition the child's activities are also limited to its area of interest. In addition, language development of the child is anomalous.

Impairment in social relationship is seen in many psychiatric disorders. Diagnosis of ASD should be made after other factors are carefully evaluated and ruled out.

NOSOLOGY

DSM-5 and ICD-10 differ in the nomenclature of ASD. This is depicted in Table 2.6.1. In the DSM-5, the disorders autism, Asperger syndrome, Rett syndrome, childhood disintegrative disorders, all have been clubbed together under the heading of ASD.

Table 2.6.1 Comparative Nosology of Autistic Spectrum Disorders

DSM-5	ICD-10
Autism Spectrum Disorder	Pervasive developmental disorders • Childhood autism • Atypical autism • Rett syndrome • Other childhood disintegrative disorder • Asperger syndrome

VIGNETTE

A 5-year-old boy was brought to the child psychiatry clinic by the parents who complained that the child was not communicating properly and was difficult to manage. The parents reported that the child did not pay attention to them since childhood and he appears to be lost in himself. He is not interested in playing with the other children. He avoids eye contact and does not answer to his name. When his parents try to play with him, he does not pay attention to their activity and does not look in the direction they are pointing to. He does not play with the toys, instead he plays with shiny articles like silver wrapper or steel utensils. He keeps rocking to and fro all by himself and at times flapping; he can continue with these activities for hours. The parents tried to get him admitted to the school but he did not interact with the teachers and other students. The child gets highly irritable in a crowded place and starts shouting and pacing around on exposure to loud noise. He likes music, which his parents use to calm him down. He was not able to go to school due to his decreased interaction and getting irritable in the classroom. Based on the history and examination, ASD was diagnosed.

CLINICAL PICTURE

The child has problem in three main areas—social relationships, language and restricted interests. The qualitative impairment in social relations is evident from early childhood. Eye contact is poorly sustained. The child does not hold up his arms in anticipation of being held. He does not appear to have interest in caregivers or other children around him. Joint attention means shared focus of two people on one object. A child of autism does not try to maintain joint attention and does not point to objects of his interest or share his experience with another person. During social interactions the child does not understand the principle of reciprocity.

In the early stage, the qualitative impairment in language is evident with lack or delay in babbling. As the child grows, he can learn some language. The communication is peculiar with inappropriate usage of words due to semantic or vocabulary errors. Echolalia, neologism and pronoun reversal may also be seen. Nonverbal communication like pointing, nodding and maintaining eye-to-eye contact are absent. The child may not answer to his name leading to the impression of having hearing impairment. Turn taking in conversation is missing. The child has also difficulty in comprehending what others are saying.

Restricted areas of interest and repetitive behaviour are routinely seen in the patients of ASD. Many children suffering from ASD are preoccupied with 'sameness' and follow the same routine daily. There may be a need to eat same food, or enter a building through the same door. Repetitive behaviour, such as hand flapping, rocking, flipping objects, lining up objects, may be seen. Occasional self-injurious behaviour, such as head banging or biting, may be seen.

The symptoms in a child may fluctuate. There may be episodes of disturbed behaviour triggered by minor variations in the daily routine or environment.

Intellectual disability is comorbid in about 70% of the patients. The prognosis is better in cases with no intellectual disability. Other common comorbidities include seizure disorder and ADHD.

NEUROBIOLOGY

Autistic spectrum disorder has many different symptoms that are governed by a variety of neural regions. However, exact neurocircuitry is yet to be understood. Brain regions that control the emotional perceptions (amygdala) and social reward circuitry (which provides us the pleasure out of social relationship), which includes extended amygdala, ventral striatum and nucleus accumbens, are involved. Besides these structures, area that is important for the facial recognition (fusiform gyrus) and those that help in interpreting the biological movements as the form of communication, eg, nodding, facial expressions, other gestures (superior temporal sulcus), are hypofunctional. Orbitofrontal cortex is important for the emotional learning and this is also having altered activity. Medial prefrontal cortex helps in social cognition and thus guides social behaviour. This has been reported to have low activity across various studies. Mirror neuron network that help us to understand the emotions of others (lateral prefrontal cortex) is also hypofunctional in ASD.

EPIDEMIOLOGY AND RISK FACTORS

The estimate of ASD is around 1 per 1000 in the population. The epidemiological studies have shown an increase in the rate of ASD in the population. This could be due to an increase in awareness in population and recognition of autistic symptoms by the clinicians. The disorder is four times more common in males.

DIFFERENCE BETWEEN ICD-10 AND DSM-5

As we have already mentioned, ICD-10 categorizes it into five major categories. In childhood autism, symptoms appear before the age of 3 years in at least one of the three areas that are described in the clinical picture. In atypical autism, symptoms appear in one of the three areas after the age of 3 years; however, all the symptoms of childhood autism are not seen.

Rett syndrome is a progressive developmental disorder found in girls. The underlying cause is mutation in the X-linked gene *MECP2*. The early development is normal with a normal head circumference. By 6–18 months, the head growth starts to decelerate, autistic symptoms emerge and growth is stagnant. The purposeful hand movements are lost and characteristic midline hand washing stereotypy is evident. The autistic symptoms may decrease with age but there is a severe mental retardation. Motor deterioration appears around the age of 10 years and the subject may be immobilized with the risk of sudden death.

Childhood disintegrative disorder is a rare disorder where the initial development is normal for the first 2 years. There is a loss of previously attained developmental milestones and autistic symptoms. The deterioration continues and then plateaus. The underlying condition in some cases may be leukodystrophies and lipidosis; in most cases no underlying cause is discernible.

Asperger syndrome is characterized by isolated deficit in social interaction in the absence of symptoms from rest of the two categories.

DIFFERENTIAL DIAGNOSIS

Severe intellectual disability may be difficult to differentiate from autism. In intellectual disability, the child makes full use of whatever language he is able to learn. The repetitive and restrictive pattern of behaviour is not evident in such patients. Nonverbal communication and social interactions are maintained in appropriate to the mental age of the patient. The repetitive behaviour needs to be differentiated from that of obsessive compulsive disorder.

Autistic symptoms may be present in the prodrome *of a psychotic disorder.* If frank hallucinations and delusions develop in the follow-up course of illness, the diagnosis may have to be revised to psychosis.

Disorders like Rett syndrome and the childhood disintegrative disorder are still categorized under ASD in ICD-10. However, these disorders have a different course and symptoms and are different from the ASD and perhaps warrant a specific diagnosis.

DIAGNOSTIC FALLACIES

Impairment in social relationship and language are seen in a number of psychiatric disorders, if only these are the core symptoms that are observed, a diagnosis of autism should be entertained.

Adults presenting for the first time in OPD may be diagnosed as having psychosis. It is essential to procure a reliable developmental history before making a diagnosis of schizophrenia if only negative symptoms are prominent.

The repetitive behaviour seen in ASD may be wrongly diagnosed as ADHD or as a behavioural disturbance with intellectual disability.

MANAGEMENT

The management of autism requires multimodal approach. The aim is to stimulate normal development of cognition, language and social relations; to decrease the maladaptive behaviour as much as possible and to decrease the burden on the family and caregiver. The core of the treatment is targeted behaviour therapy targeting individual behaviour. The caregiver's education and training is an essential part of the management. Medication is ineffective in the core symptoms but may be given to patients with unmanageable behavioural disturbances.

COURSE AND PROGNOSIS

The progression of symptom varies in each patient. Outcome depends on the intelligence and ability to communicate. Some patients are able to adapt and communicate effectively; they may be involved in some vocational activities under supervision or even independently. Others continue to require constant care and supervision. Learning and compensation continue throughout life.

SUMMARY

- ASD are a group of neurodevelopmental disorders.
- The disorders are characterized by qualitative impairment in social relations, qualitative reduction in language and restricted and repetitive behaviour.
- The severity in impairment often correlates with the acquisition of language and severity of comorbid intellectual disability.
- An early intervention with targeted behaviour therapy may improve the outcome.

FURTHER READING

1. American Psychiatric Association. (2013). "Diagnostic and Statistical Manual of Mental Disorders." 5th edit, Author, Washington, DC.
2. Maximo J. O., Cadena E. J., and Kana R. K. (2014). The Implication of Brain Connectivity in Neuropsychology of Autism, *Neuropsychology Review*, 24:16–31.
3. World Health Organization. (1992). "The ICD-10 Classification of Mental and Behavioural Disorders: Clinical Descriptions and Diagnostic Guidelines." Author, Geneva.

TIC DISORDERS

Ravi Gupta

Tic disorder is characterized by repeated and nonrhythmic movements of a part of the body or vocalizations that appear suddenly and last for a short period. These activities are involuntary in nature.

NOSOLOGY

The nomenclature of tic disorders differs between DSM-5 and ICD-10 as shown in Table 2.7.1.

VIGNETTE

A 10-year-old boy was brought with complaints of making some abnormal shrugging movements for the past 1 year. He also sometimes makes grunting sound. These vocalizations and shrugging movement appear out of context and recur multiple times a day. These movements increase during stress but are not limited to the periods of heightened anxiety. These movements are sudden and last for a second or so. The child is usually unaware of these movements and vocalizations. The family members and teachers forbid him from doing so and, at that time, he could transiently control them, but they appear again.

CLINICAL PICTURE

Tics can be simple or complex. Simple motor tics include shrugging, eye blinking or moving any of the limbs. Simple vocal tics include throat clearing, moaning and sniffing.

Table 2.7.1 Comparative Nosology of Tic Disorders

DSM-5	ICD-10
Tourett disorder	Combined vocal and multiple motor tic disorder (de la Tourett syndrome)
Persistent vocal or motor tic disorder	Chronic vocal or motor tic disorder
Provisional tic disorder	Transient tic disorders

Table 2.7.2 Comparison of Tic Disorders

	Tourett Disorder	Persistent Motor or Vocal Tic Disorder	Provisional Tic Disorder
Tics	Motor and vocal both must be present	Either motor or vocal tics	Either motor or vocal tics
Age of onset	Before 18 years	Before 18 years	Before 18 years
Duration	At least 1 year since the first tic onset	At least 1 year since the first tic onset	Less than 1 year since the first tic onset
Exclude	Cocaine use disorder, Huntington disease, postviral encephalitis		

On the other hand, complex motor tics last for a longer duration and they involve more than one muscle group,eg, head turning with shoulder shrugging. Especially troublesome complex motor tics are copropraxia (making obscene sexual gesture) or imitating other's movements (echopraxia). These may sometimes appear as normal movements but their repeated occurrence and involuntary nature differentiate them from voluntary movements. Similarly, complex vocal tics include producing a legible sound, eg, repeating own words (palilaia), repetition of other's words or phrase (echolalia) and sometimes socially inappropriate words (coprolalia). The patients report a feeling of mounting tension when they are forbidden to do so or try to control it themselves. For the diagnosis of Tourett disorder, both vocal as well as motor tics must be evident. This disorder is called persistent if the symptoms last for more than 1 year. It must be considered that this disorder may run a relapsing-remitting course, so, in the history, there may be some periods that are free of any kind of tic. The patients have partial control over tics and they can suppress them for varying periods. Table 2.7.2 compares the disorders that are covered under the rubric of tic disorders.

NEUROBIOLOGY

An increased activity in the ventral and midline striatum is considered the locus of the pathology in tic disorders. In addition, higher activity has been found in the orbitofrontal cortex and motor cortex.

This disorder may arise because of a congenital dysfunction in the neuronal movement as parvalbumin-expressing neurons have been found in lesser number in the dorsal striatum and in higher number in the globus pallidus in these patients. In normal situations, the opposite is seen.

In addition, in the dorsal striatum, another type of cells, cholinergic tonically active neurons have been found to be reduced. Normally, these neurons reduce the dopamine in the striatum. Reduction in the number of these neurons in these patients is associated with an enhanced dopaminergic tone, which can lead to the development of tic disorder.

EPIDEMIOLOGY AND RISK FACTORS

Estimated prevalence of Tourett disorder is between 0.3% to 0.8% of school children. Males are affected more as compared to females.

Table 2.7.3 Differences in ICD-10 as Compared to DSM-5		
Tourett Disorder	**Persistent Motor or Vocal Tic Disorder**	**Provisional Tic Disorder**
ICD-10 states that period of remission should not be more than 2 months between two episodes	ICD-10 states that period of remission should not be more than 2 months between two episodes	Tics must be present for at least 1 month

COMPARISON OF ICD-10 AND DSM-5 SYMPTOMATOLOGY

ICD-10 has some differences from the DSM-5 in description of symptomatology. This is outlined in Table 2.7.3.

DIFFERENTIAL DIAGNOSIS

Tics must be differentiated from the stereotyped movements. Stereotyped movements are purposeful and include finger wriggling and waving of hands. They last for longer duration and patients do not complain of 'mounting tension' as reported before the tic. Stereotypes movements exacerbate when the person is engaged deeply into any activity, eg, thinking and reading, and cease when the person is distracted.

Rapid, random, irregular, jerky, continuous, repetitive and sometimes bilateral movements characterize chorea. It must be differentiated from tics.

They must be differentiated from dyskinesias that are precipitated by voluntary movements and exertion.

Myoclonus is a sudden jerky movement in one direction and cannot be suppressed. These movements are not rhythmic.

Tics must be differentiated from obsessive–compulsive disorder.

DIAGNOSTIC FALLACIES

Some people have some habitual movements, eg, continuously moving their legs while sitting or any other movement (scratching the head while thinking). These should not be diagnosed as tic disorder as these movements are not associated with a sense of tension, even if the subjects are forbidden in doing so.

MANAGEMENT

Since the dopaminergic tone is high in tic disorders, use of dopamine antagonists, eg, antipsychotics, are useful in the management of tic disorders. Usually, high potency antipsychotics, eg, haloperidol (0.5–20 mg/day) or risperidone (0.5–16 mg/day) are given. Another class of medication that has been found effective is alpha-2-agonists, eg, clonidine (0.05–0.5 mg/day) and guanfacine (0.5–4 mg/day). In intractable cases, injections of botulinum toxin may be used.

Behavioural techniques, eg, 'exposure and response prevention' and self monitoring have been tried. However, among all the behavioural techniques, currently we have sufficient evidences regarding the efficacy of habit reversal training (HRT) only.

COURSE AND PROGNOSIS

These disorders run a waxing–waning course. Most of the patients of tic disorder are children and with the increment in age, this disorder usually improves. Only a minority of patients have symptoms during adulthood.

SUMMARY

- Tic disorders are common among children and adolescents.
- Tics originate because of the abnormality in corticostriatal circuitry.
- Antipsychotics are useful in the management of tics.

FURTHER READING

1. American Psychiatric Association. (2013). "Diagnostic and Statistical Manual of Mental Disorders." 5th edit, Author, Washington, DC.
2. Bloch M., State M., and Pittenger C. (2011). Recent Advances in Tourett Syndrome, *Current Opinion in Neurology*, 24:119–125.
3. Frank M., and Cavanna A. E. (2013). Behavioural Treatments for Tourette Syndrome: An Evidence-Based Review. *Behavioural Neurology*, 27:105–117.
4. Shprecher D., and Kurlan R. (2009). The Management of Tics. *Movement Disorders*, 24:15–24.
5. World Health Organization. (1992). "The ICD-10 Classification of Mental and Behavioural Disorders: Clinical Descriptions and Diagnostic Guidelines." Author, Geneva.

MOOD DISORDERS

3.1

Ravi Gupta

Mood disorders are characterized by a disturbance in the mood. Mood can be defined as an emotional feeling tone that is pervasive and long lasting and it colours the life of a person. This means that mood is an emotional state that lasts for some days to some months and it influences a whole gamut of behaviours and feelings.

Phasic changes in the mood may be seen within a given time period; however, these should not be relied upon while making the diagnosis of a mood disorder. Normally, our mood fluctuates within a small spectrum; however, mood disorders are diagnosed when the mood disturbance crosses these limits and persist for a defined period. Though the mood state may vary from apathy, anxiety, irritability to depressed and euphoric to exalted mood, still, classically in mood disorders we consider only two kinds of fluctuations—one is persistent sadness of mood (depression) and the other is elation of mood (mania) or an alteration between them. DSM-5 has separated the depression from bipolar disorders owing to different neurobiological underpinnings. We will follow the same concept in this chapter and first we will discuss about the depression and subsequently about the bipolar disorder.

3.1.1 DEPRESSIVE DISORDERS

These disorders are characterized by persistent and pervasive sad mood, along with other symptoms, for a defined period. The duration of symptoms helps us to determine a specific depressive disorder.

NOSOLOGY

Refer Table 3.1.1.1.

Table 3.1.1.1 Comparative Nosology of Depressive Disorders	
DSM-5	**ICD-10**
Disruptive mood dysregulation disorder	_____
Major depressive disorder	
Single episode	Depressive episode
Recurrent episode	Recurrent depressive disorder
Persistent depressive disorder	Dysthymia
Premenstrual dysphoric disorder	–

VIGNETTE

A 27-year-old female presented with complaints of sadness of mood for the past 1 month. She reported that she has lost interest in all the activities that were previously pleasurable to her. She now feels sad for most of the day and is not able to perform her duties. She has noticed a reduction in sleep with multiple nocturnal awakenings. Sometimes, she wakes up early in the morning, way ahead of her usual waking time and then she is unable to fall asleep. She has lost her appetite since 1 month and now she does not feel like eating. She also reported a change in her thoughts in a way that she had developed a negative approach towards life. Her thoughts are often pessimistic and prevent her from starting any new work. She often feels helpless and as if she has been trapped inside a cocoon, which she would never be able to break. She also had a similar episode 3 years back that responded well to the pharmacological treatment. General physical examination did not add anything to the diagnosis. On mental status examination, she showed psychomotor retardation, slow speech, short answers, sad mood and affect along with depressive thoughts. Based on the history and examination, a diagnosis of major depressive disorder with recurrent episodes, currently major depressive episode was made and treatment was started.

CLINICAL PICTURE

Largely, the symptoms of depression may be catalogued into four categories—mood, psychomotor activity, biological functions and cognitive symptoms.

When asked about the mood, patients with depressive disorders mainly complain of persistent sadness of mood and no activity is able to bring any amount of pleasure to them except for a brief period. They also lose interest in all the activities that were pleasurable to them earlier, eg, a person may say that earlier he enjoyed watching television, but now does not feel any pleasure in doing so, or a person who was always fond of listening to music has lost the inclination towards music since the onset of illness. Sometimes, especially among adolescents, irritable mood may be reported instead of sad mood.

A change in the psychomotor activity may be seen with psychomotor retardation and they often spend whole day sitting at one place or lying in bed for prolonged periods. Their movements become slow (bradykinesia), which may sometimes go up to the level of negative catatonia.

A change in the biological functions may be seen with sleep disturbances, reduced appetite and loss of libido. However, in cases of atypical depression, sleep, appetite and libido may be increased.

These symptoms are associated with cognitive complaints, eg, poor concentration, memory lapses and difficulty in taking decisions. They often have pessimistic thoughts and report a feeling of hopelessness (things will never be right) and helplessness (nobody can help me). They lose self-confidence and have a negative view of themselves. They feel that they will not be able to do anything and often convey inability to do petty tasks that they used to do easily during asymptomatic period (Fig. 3.1.1.1). Interference in the personal, social and occupational functioning is reported because of the symptoms.

These disorders may be categorized into various subtypes depending upon the age of onset, duration of episode, severity of illness and ancillary symptoms (Table 3.1.1.2).

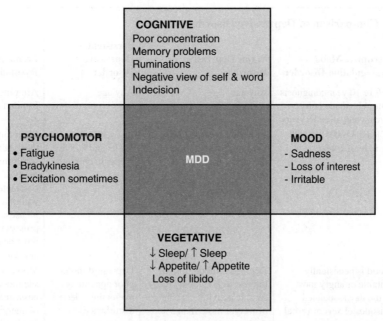

FIGURE 3.1.1.1.

Symptom dimensions in depressive disorders.

NEUROBIOLOGY

Neurobiology of the depressive disorder has been hypothesized to link with stress, which has been considered to evoke a depressive episode in genetically predisposed people. However, it must be remembered that in a group of patients, it may develop even without stress. For such cases, it has been argued that they have such high genetic predisposition (if we would ever be able to quantify it) that a trivial stress, too insignificant to get noticed, can evoke depressive disorder. To make the issue more complex, you should appreciate the fact that stress is ubiquitous and even if I ask you to think about the stressful moments during the past 24 h, you will be able to name a few that you have experienced (please refer to Chapter 3.6 for details). Thus, the linkage between the two may be over-simplistic and spurious as well. Leaving this debate here, we will focus on our current understanding of the neurobiology of depression.

Current concepts state that a stress (or some other yet to be discovered stimulus) activates hypothalamic–pituitary–adrenal (HPA) axis after being provoked by the prefrontal cortex and amygdala. Stimulation of the HPA axis results in the release of cortisol, which further activates the amygdala. Thus, the HPA axis and amygdala work in a feed-forward manner to activate each other. However, this activity is checked by another arm that involves hippocampus. Cortisol stimulates the hippocampus, which in turn, sends inhibitory signals to the HPA axis to contain its activity.

Activity of the HPA axis is not only dependent upon the neuroanatomical area but also by the type of signals emerging from some of the area. Emotional self-regulation (see 'Cognitive Behaviour Therapy' in Chapter 9.1) limits the activity of the HPA axis by altering the activity in the prefrontal and limbic areas.

Table 3.1.1.2 Comparison of Depressive Disorders

	Disruptive Mood Dysregulation Disorder	Major Depressive Disorder	Persistent Depressive Disorder	Premenstrual Dysphoric Dsisorder
Age of onset	Before 10 years;diagnosis cannot be made before 6 years and after 18 years	Any age	Any age	After menarche. Limited to women
Frequency and duration	At least 3 times a week for at least 1 year	At least 2 weeks; symptoms are present most of the days for almost every day	At least 2 years in adults and at least 1 year in children	Symptoms appear a week before menses, start improving with onset of menses and completely resolve within a week after menses;diagnosis is prospective; symptoms must be present during at least two cycles
Symptoms	Mood is persistently irritable or angry most of the day;associated episodes of severe verbal or physical aggression that is out of proportion to the provocation	Depressed mood, loss of interest in previously pleasurable activities, a change of weight more than 5% (loss or gain), altered sleep, loss of energy, feelings of worthlessness, cognitive disturbances, recurrent thoughts of harming oneself	Depressed mood, poor appetite or overeating, sleep disturbances (increased or decreased), fatigue, low self-esteem, impaired concentration, hopelessness	Mood swings, irritable, sad mood, hopelessness, anxiety, lack of energy, reduced interest in daily activities, lethargy, weight gain, breast tenderness, disturbances in sleep and appetite
Exclude	Depressive disorder and mania	Bereavement, natural disaster, serious medical illness or any other disability (see diagnostic fallacies)	–	–

Relative activity of these areas decides the activity of the HPA axis that is responsible for subsequent processes, like changes in neurotransmission, neuronal damage and release of inflammatory markers (please refer to Chapter 3.6). High activity of the HPA axis causes neuronal damage in hippocampal area. It results in the loss of hippocampal volume and, at the functional level, reduces control over the activity of the HPA axis. Similar neuronal damage has also been observed in the prefrontal cortex during high activity of the HPA axis.

To master a stressful situation, we have two distinct but interacting circuits in the brain. First, the ventral circuit regulates emotions and it includes amygdala, ventral striatum, anterior hippocampus, insula, subgenual anterior cingulate cortex and orbito–frontal cortex; and second, the dorsal cognitive circuit includes posterior hippocampus, pregenual part of anterior cingulate cortex and dorsolateral prefrontal cortex (Fig. 3.1.1.2). Ventral pathway is instrumental in dealing with emotional stimuli, providing them an emotional salience and autonomic regulation, whereas the dorsal circuit is important in executive functioning, decision making, memory, attention, planning and, lastly, regulation of ventral circuit. In normal situations, dorsal circuit regulates the activity of the ventral circuit. However, in depression, because of low activity of the hippocampus (see above), activity of the dorsal circuit decreases, resulting in heightened

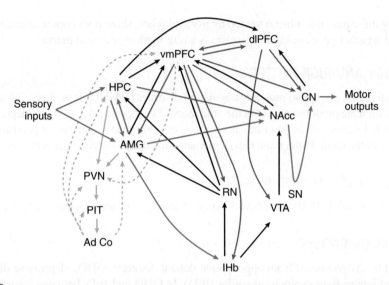

FIGURE 3.1.1.2

Neuronal circuits in depressive disorders. dIPFC, dorsolateral prefrontal cortex; vmPFC, ventromedial prefrontal cortex; HPC, hippocampus; AMG, amygdala; PVN, paraventricular nuclei; PIT, pituitary; AdCo, adrenal cortex; IHb, lateral hebenula; RN, raphe nuclei; VTA, ventral tegmental area; SN, substantia nigra; NAcc, nucleus accumbens; CN, caudate nucleus.

(Reproduced with permission from: Willner P, Scheel-Krügerb J, Belzungc C. The neurobiology of depression and antidepressant action. Neurosci Biobehav Rev 2013;37(10):2331–2371.)

activity in the ventral circuit. Thus, in depressive disorders, activity of the ventral circuit increases, whereas that of the dorsal circuit is diminished, resulting in mood (sadness, anxiety, depressive ruminations) and cognitive symptoms (eg, psychomotor retardation, apathy, attention and memory disturbances).

Release of cortisol also reduces the dopamine release in nucleus accumbens, which receives dopaminergic fibres from ventral tegmental area (VTA) and is important for the feeling of reward. However, this reduction is seen only during pleasurable stimuli, but not during painful stimuli. This is why depressed patients do not have the feeling of pleasure, but have intact feelings of pain and punishment. Furthermore, the activity of the VTA is regulated by the prefrontal cortex and hippocampus and a reduction in activity (secondary to neuronal damage as mentioned above) in these areas may lead to reduced dopamine availability in nucleus accumbens. This compounds the situation further.

Hebenula is also instrumental in this mechanism. Its activity is increased during stress that leads to enhanced appreciation of negative stimulus (via the activation of serotonergic neurons in the raphe nuclei (RN) that are supplied to amygdala), whereas reduced feeling of positive events via inhibition of VTA dopamine neurons that terminate in nucleus accumbens. Note that amygdala has connections with the hypothalamus as well and these connections could be responsible for the vegetative symptoms of depression.

Psychological literature says that these patients are not able to cope with stress. This ability of coping is also dependent upon the relative activity of the ventral and dorsal circuits, in addition to the activity of amygdala and nucleus accumbens. Changes akin to those described above are seen when a person considers any situation as negative, even momentarily (*There is nothing psychological!*). This could be one reason why these patients, when assessed by psychologists, show poor coping mechanisms. This is yet to be found whether poor coping mechanism is a trait marker or a state marker.

EPIDEMIOLOGY AND RISK FACTORS

One year prevalence of disruptive mood dysregulation disorder (DMDD) is between 2% and 5% in the United States with male predominance. On the other hand, 1 year prevalence of major depressive episode is 7% in the United States with higher rates among women. One year prevalence of persistent depressive disorder is 0.5% in the United States and that of premenstrual dysphoric disorder is between 2% and 6%.

COMPARISON OF ICD-10 AND DSM-5

Differences between the ICD-10 and DSM-5 symptomatology are presented in Table 3.1.1.3.

DIFFERENTIAL DIAGNOSIS

DMDD should be differentiated from oppositional defiant disorder (ODD), depressive disorder, bipolar disorder and intermittent explosive disorder (IED). In ODD and IED, between disruptive episodes mood remains euthymic. Bipolar disorders have history of mania or hypomania. Patients with depressive disorder do not have recurrent aggression as seen in DMDD.

Major depressive disorder must be differentiated from bipolar disorder and attention deficit hyperactivity disorder by the absence of manic symptoms and absence of typical attention deficit hyperactivity disorder (ADHD) symptoms.

Persistent depressive disorder must be differentiated from major depressive disorder by the duration of symptoms and episodic course.

Premenstrual dysphoric disorder must be differentiated from dysmenorrhoea and bipolar disorders by the absence of pain and manic episodes, respectively.

DIAGNOSTIC FALLACIES

1. Clinical picture after bereavement or financial loss or after any other major stressor may be similar to that of major depressive disorder. In those cases, diagnosis of major depressive episode should be made carefully. If ruminations regarding the loss, inability to take appropriate measures to prevent the mishap that has occurred and self-derogatory ideas dominate the clinical picture, diagnosis of major depressive episode should be deferred unless the person has feelings of worthlessness, and poor self-esteem. In these cases, death-wish or suicidal ideation arises because of the inability to cope with the situation rather than the feelings of 'I am not worth living' or 'I do not deserve to live anymore' or an inability to cope with the depression (as seen in major depressive episode).

Table 3.1.1.3 Difference in ICD-10 from DSM-5			
Disruptive Mood Dysregulation Disorder	**Major Depressive Disorder**	**Persistent Depressive Disorder**	**Premenstrual Dysphoric Disorder**
Not included in ICD-10	No difference	Almost similar	Not included in ICD-10

2. Patients with chronic insomnia, chronically poor-quality sleep (secondary to restless legs syndrome, obstructive sleep apnoea) and insufficient sleep syndrome often present with daytime symptoms that overlap those of depressive disorders. Most of these patients improve with resolution of underlying sleep problems without the antidepressants. In these cases, mood is reported to be 'tired' or 'lethargic' instead of 'sad'. Similarly, these cases lack other mood symptoms.

3. Chronic fatigue syndrome grossly overlaps the clinical picture of depression. However, in these cases as well, mood is reported to be 'fatigued' rather than sad.

MANAGEMENT

The mainstay of management for the moderate to severe depressive episodes is pharmacotherapy. However, cases with mild severity may be amenable to the *structured* cognitive behaviour therapy. For pharmacotherapy, we have a number of antidepressants that belong to different classes. Choice of drug depends upon the clinical picture (some symptoms respond better to dopaminergic, whereas others to serotonergic or noradrenergic drugs), adverse effect profile of the drug, prior response to the therapy and other medical conditions. In some cases, addition of benzodiazepine may be required to control the anxiety.

Commonly used drugs and their doses are listed in Table 3.1.1.4.

In some cases, you may find associated medical morbidities, eg, congestive heart failure or diabetes mellitus. Patients with severe depression are often not able to comply with the prescribed management for these illnesses leading to a life-threatening situation. Similarly, suicidal thoughts also pose a threat to life, necessitating the urgent treatment of depression. In all such cases, modified electroconvulsive therapy (mECT) becomes the treatment of choice, provided it is not contraindicated, for the fact that it improves the illness at a faster rate. It is also the treatment of choice for depression during pregnancy. mECT should preferably be administered after admitting the patient. Similarly, patients who are not taking food because of depression should be admitted to provide the supportive therapy (feeding through nasogastric tube and parenteral fluids). Patients with compliance issues related to antidepressant therapy should also be admitted to ensure drug compliance.

COURSE AND PROGNOSIS

Course of major depressive disorder is variable. Some patients have just one episode, whereas others may have recurrent episodes. Each episode increases the chances of having subsequent episode and poor response to therapy. Hence, each episode must be treated energetically.

Table 3.1.1.4 Commonly used Antidepressants

Name	Dose	Common Adverse Effects
Classical antidepressants		
Imipramine	25–150 mg/day	Anticholinergic adverse effects, sedation
Clomipramine	25–150 mg/day	Anticholinergic adverse effects, sedation
Newer antidepressants		
Fluoxetine	20–80 mg/day	Anxiety, reduced appetite, delayed ejaculation
Sertraline	50–200 mg/day	Anxiety, reduced appetite, delayed ejaculation
Bupropion	150–450 mg/day	Seizures beyond 300 mg/day
Vialzodone	10–40 mg/day	Anxiety
Mirtazepine	15–60mg/day	Sedation, increased appetite

SUMMARY

- Depressive disorders constitute one of the most prevalent psychiatric disorders.
- They arise because of neurobiological disturbances.
- They mimic a number of conditions, thus, increasing the chances of false positive diagnosis.
- Antidepressants are effective in their management.

3.1.2 BIPOLAR DISORDERS

Bipolar disorders are characterized by change in the mood with episodes of elated mood with or without intermittent major depressive disorder. In these cases, depressive episode may be subtle and short-lasting that may gone unnoticed; hence, documentation of depressive episode is not required. Fig. 3.1.2.1 shows the longitudinal change in mood in a normal person during depressive disorders and among patients with bipolar disorders. Before going further, we need to understand the nosology of bipolar disorders.

NOSOLOGY

Classification of bipolar disorders according to DSM-5 and ICD-10 is depicted in Table 3.1.2.1.

VIGNETTE

A 23–year–old boy was brought by the family members because he was not behaving normally. According to his family members, the behavioural changes started appearing 20 days back; however, since the past 10 days, the symptoms have turned more severe. They noticed that he has started considering himself a very important person who could make a big discovery. However, when they asked him about the project, he could not provide them with any satisfactory reply. He had started spending money without any reasons and donated his bike to a person whom he saw tired and walking on the road. His mood was elated and he appeared overtly cheerful without any reason. He started wearing fancy clothes that were inappropriate to the occasions. His socialization also increased and at times he was found giving speech in the neighbourhood about bringing a revolution. His speech output had increased and he kept on talking for hours without any apparent context. A change in the content of his speech had also been observed, as mentioned above. He finds it difficult to sit at one place and keeps on moving. He hardly sleeps for an hour each night and he spends rest of the night reading. When he was forbidden by the family members for some of these activities, he became irritated and blamed that they could not understand why he has taken the birth in this world. Physical examination did not reveal anything significant. However, his mental status examination disclosed poor concentration, increased psychomotor activity, elated mood, flight of ideas and delusion of grandiosity. Based on the history and examination, diagnosis of manic episode was made.

CLINICAL PICTURE

Contrary to depressive disorders, clinical picture in manic phase of bipolar disorder is dominated by the euphoric or excessively cheerful mood. This is associated with feelings of grandiosity and increased

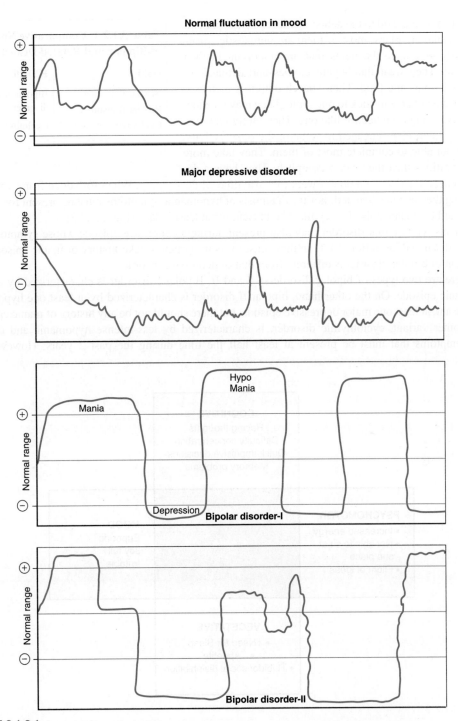

FIGURE 3.1.2.1

Longitudinal change in mood in a normal person, during depressive disorders and in bipolar disorders.

self-esteem that are up to the delusional level. These patients always make big plans, most of them are unrealistic, spend recklessly or donate the items that are important in their daily life. They wear flamboyant clothes and demand for expensive items and food. Their speech output is increased but they are not able to stick to one topic. They may consider themselves kings and behave like one. They rarely feel tired and keep themselves engaged in some or the other activity, but are not able to complete most of them. They take more responsibilities than they can accomplish. They have a decreased need for sleep and do not want to waste time while sleeping. When forbidden from what they are doing they become irritated. For the diagnosis of hypomania, symptoms must be present for at least 4 days and for manic episode they must be present for at least 7 days (Fig. 3.1.2.2).

Table 3.1.2.1 Comparative Nosology of Bipolar and Related Disorders	
DSM-5	ICD-10
Bipolar I disorder	Bipolar affective disorder
Bipolar II disorder	
Cyclothymic disorder	Cyclothymia

Patients with bipolar disorder may also present during a depressive episode whose symptoms are already discussed in section 3.1.1. In these cases it is important to take history of manic episodes, as treatment of bipolar disorder is different from that of depressive disorder.

There are two types of bipolar disorders—I and II. Bipolar I disorder is characterized by at least one manic episode. On the other hand, bipolar II disorder is characterized by at least one hypomanic episode and at least one major depressive episode, but there should not be any history of manic episode.

Another variant, cyclothymic disorder, is characterized by less-intense hypomanic and depressive symptoms that must be present at least half the time during the past 2 years. However, the

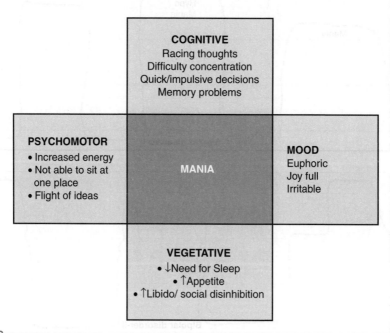

FIGURE 3.1.2.2

Symptom dimensions of mania.

severity of symptoms should not reach to the level of hypomania, mania or major depressive disorder (Fig. 3.1.2.1).

These symptoms interfere with the personal, social and occupational functioning of the patient.

NEUROBIOLOGY

The neurobiological pathways in bipolar disorder have not been analysed in detail owing to difficulty in performing functional neuroimaging during manic state. A decreased activity has been observed in inferior frontal gyrus that signifies impulsivity seen during mania. Reduction in the activity of the amygdala has also been observed, but this is inconsistent across studies.

EPIDEMIOLOGY

One-year prevalence of bipolar I disorder is 0.6% with a slight male dominance, whereas that of bipolar II disorder is 0.3%.

DIFFERENCE BETWEEN DSM-5 AND ICD-10

Diagnostic criteria are almost similar between the two classifications except the fact that ICD-10 does not classify bipolar disorder into separate categories and considers it as the part of mood disorder.

DIFFERENTIAL DIAGNOSIS

These disorders must be differentiated from one another and from depressive disorders based on the symptoms of all the episodes and duration as well as severity of symptoms.

One important differential diagnosis is attention deficit hyperactivity disorder that may have symptoms that are similar to mania, except the fact that mood remains euthymic in ADHD and symptoms are continuous. Moreover, in ADHD, symptoms are present since childhood.

These disorders must be differentiated from borderline personality disorder as the latter have it's onset during adolescence and have continuous course of symptoms. Cyclothymic disorder, in particular, may be difficult to differentiate from borderline personality disorder.

DIAGNOSTIC FALLACIES

1. Transient changes in the mood (both euphoria and depression) that are not sufficient to induce any dysfunction are common and should not be mistaken for bipolar disorders.
2. A number of substances, especially stimulants and some drugs, eg, steroids, l-dopa or antidepressants, may induce symptoms akin to mania. In these cases, adequate wash-out period should be given and if symptoms persist after the termination of physiological effect of that substance then only diagnosis of bipolar disorder should be made.

MANAGEMENT

Mainstay of the treatment is mood stabilizers that are chosen on the basis of history of mood disorder, target symptom, previous response to the therapy and adverse effects. Lithium carbonate

(300–900 mg/day) and valproate (up to 25 mg/kg per day) may be prescribed. At times, antipsychotics are necessary, especially for the management of delusions. Antidepressants may be required during depressive episodes depending upon the clinical history. Mirtazepine and bupropion are considered safer as they have fewer propensities to induce mania.

However, patients who are a threat to their own safety or to the others because of their symptoms are the candidates for admission. Similarly, if there is any compromise to the existence of life because of associated medical comorbidities, admission is required. In such cases, chemical restriction (drug-induced extra pyramidal syndrome [EPS] and sedation) to curtail the psychomotor activity may be tried using high potency antipsychotics in large doses (eg, 5 mg haloperidol every 30 min oral or parenteral in the maximum tolerable dose) with or without benzodiazepines. mECT may also be used to curtail the psychomotor activity.

COURSE AND PROGNOSIS

This disease often has the relapsing and remitting course with complete recovery in-between.

SUMMARY

- Bipolar disorders have episodes of mania and depression.
- Manic episodes show symptoms that are just opposite of depression.

FURTHER READING

Depressive Disorders

1. American Psychiatric Association. (2013). "Diagnostic and Statistical Manual of Mental Disorders." 5th edit, Author, Washington, DC.
2. Willner P., Scheel-Krüger J., and Belzung C. (2013). The Neurobiology of Depression and Antidepressant Action. *Neuroscience &Biobehavioral Reviews*, 37:2331–2371.
3. World Health Organization. (1992). "The ICD-10 Classification of Mental and Behavioral Disorders: Clinical Descriptions and Diagnostic Guidelines."Author, Geneva.

Bipolar Disorders

1. American Psychiatric Association. (2013). "Diagnostic and Statistical Manual of Mental Disorders." 5th edit, Author, Washington, DC.
2. Chen C. H., Suckling J., Lennox B. R., Ooi C., and Bullmore E. T. (2011). A Quantitative Meta-analysis of fMRI Studies in Bipolar Disorder. *Bipolar Disorders*, 13:1–15.
3. World Health Organization. (1992). "The ICD-10 Classification of Mental and Behavioural Disorders: Clinical Descriptions and Diagnostic Guidelines."Author, Geneva.

SCHIZOPHRENIA AND OTHER PSYCHOTIC DISORDERS

3.2

Ravi Gupta

Conceptually, psychotic disorders are congenital abnormalities in the microstructure of cortex culminating in dysfunctional cortical glutaminergic–GABAergic neurotransmission that in turn leads to functional changes in the dopaminergic neurotransmission to produce a clinical syndrome.

Clinically, they present having perceptual problems (hallucinations), thought disorders (loosening of association and delusions) and gross abnormal behaviours, like collecting garbage without any reason and inappropriate giggling. In addition, motor problems (eg, excessive motor activity or stuporous catatonia), mood disturbance (eg, anxiety, fear and elation) and cognitive disturbances (eg, poor attention, concentration, memory changes, poor reasoning and abstraction) are also seen.

In this chapter, we will discuss the pathophysiology, diagnosis and management of these disorders.

NOSOLOGY

DSM-5 and ICD-10 systems classify these disorders differently, as depicted in Table 3.2.1.

Table 3.2.1 Comparative Nosology of Psychotic Disorders

DSM-5	ICD-10
Schizotypal (personality) disorder	Schizotypal disorder
Brief psychotic disorder	Acute and transient psychotic disorder
Schizophreniform disorder	–
Schizophrenia	Schizophrenia
Schizoaffective disorder	Schizoaffective disorder
Delusional disorder	Persistent delusional disorder
Catatonia associated with mental or medical disorder	–
Unspecified schizophrenia spectrum and other psychotic disorder	Psychosis not otherwise specified

VIGNETTE

A 23-year-old male was brought by his family members. The family members reported that his behaviour has changed around 8 months back. Initially, the symptoms were mild but progressed gradually and he became unmanageable at home during the past 1 month. He does not sleep at all, keeps muttering as if talking to somebody whom others cannot see and is not able to take care of himself. He has a firm belief that family members want to kill him and does not eat anything at home. Out of this fear, he had called police twice in the past 3 days for help. He was an engineer working in a multinational company but now he is not able to attend to his work. Sometimes he scribbles in the notebook and writes some letters that nobody seems to understand. He stopped attending social gatherings because he feels that people talk about him and they are planning to kill him. There was no history to suggest any neurological disorder, consumption of substances of abuse or any drug ingestion. Family history was negative for any psychiatric disorder.

On examination, he appeared conscious and oriented. He had poor personal hygiene and was stinking. He was poorly clad and kempt. He was smiling without any reason and muttering. He appeared to be distracted by trivial stimuli in the surroundings. When he was asked as to why he was not eating food, he reported that the family members were actually conspiring against him so that they could snatch his property. Despite presenting contradictory evidences, he stood firm on this idea. He claimed to have a connection with the God who talks to him in three different voices. He reported that the 'God' directed him to do all the activities that he was doing.

Based on the history and symptoms, diagnosis of schizophrenia was made and treatment was initiated.

CLINICAL PICTURE

Clinically, symptoms and signs of schizophrenia spectrum and other psychotic disorders can be divided into five different domains: (a) positive symptoms; (b) negative symptoms; (c) mood changes; (d) cognitive symptoms; (e) aggression and impulsivity.

Positive symptoms are those that are not a part of normal behaviour and are superimposed upon it during the symptomatic period. These include perceptual disturbances, ie, hallucinations, and thought disorders, eg, delusions.

Auditory hallucinations are the hallmark of psychotic disorders, although other hallucinations can be reported, except for visual hallucinations that are extremely rare in this condition. Most often, the patient reports that two or more people are talking to each other and he/she is listening to them as the third party (*third person hallucinations*); or that somebody talks to him/her directly and asks him/her to do something (*commanding hallucinations*); or that somebody gives a running commentary onhis/her actions (*running commentary type*). Rarely, they may report that their thoughts are audible to them and they can hear whatever comes to their mind (*thought echo*).

Thought abnormalities are not rare and these patients present with delusions. Most common type of delusions that we see in these patients are that of paranoid type (Fig. 3.2.1). However, at times, grandiose delusions can also be seen. Sometimes, delusions are weird and appear impossible and implausible, known as bizarre delusions, eg, a female patient may say that somebody from the Mars raped her and that she is carrying his child. Another idea could be that some international agency is

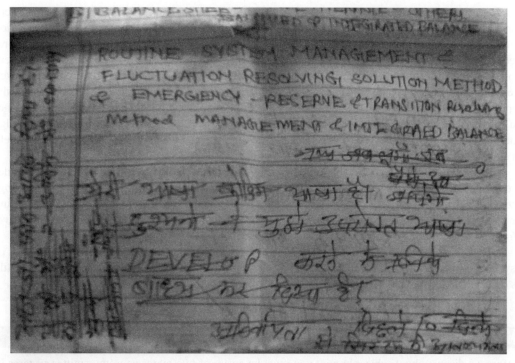

FIGURE 3.2.1

Letter from a patient of schizophrenia during symptomatic period showing loosening of association and delusion of persecution.

(Source: *Himalayan Hospital, Dehradun*).

spying on the patient, even when he appears to have a low-priority job. The cultural background and patient's knowledge and exposure to technology influence bizarreness of the idea.

They sometimes feel that people come to know about their thoughts or that their thoughts are being broadcasted (*thought broadcasting*) or that people are inserting their (people's) thoughts in them (*thought insertion*). This may increase to the feeling where they sense that other people can control their emotions (*make affect*) or can regulate their activity (*make volition*) and they feel that they are the puppets in the hands of others (*passivity phenomenon*). Sometimes they may communicate that their thoughts have been withdrawn and they are not able to think (*thought withdrawal*).

Sometimes these patients present with **negative symptoms** and they appear indifferent to surroundings (*apathy*). They may lose interest in daily activities (*anhedonia*) and do nothing at all (*avolition*). They stop paying social visits (*asocialisation*) and do not have the motivation to talk to anybody (*abulia*). Sometimes, motor activity is so reduced that these patients become stuporous (*catatonic*). Patients with catatonia show a variety of symptoms, eg, *psychogenic pillow* (eg, they keep their head in the air, even when the pillow is removed), *waxy flexibility* (they behave as if their body is made up of wax and the examiner is able to change its posture without any resistance), *posturing* (maintain the posture for hours that they are left in). They may follow commands automatically without showing any resistance (*automatic obedience*).

Cognitive symptoms are common among these patients and perhaps the main reason behind poor functioning. They show problems with working memory, declarative memory, attention, concentration and reasoning. They have abnormality in filtering the unwanted stimuli. These abnormalities are reflected as problems in making decisions in day-to-day life and negatively affect the functioning. Attention problems also influence the thinking and these patients often lose the train of thought and switch from one to other issue inappropriately (*loss of association or incoherence*) or sometimes they lose the topic they were talking about and start talking something new abruptly (*thought block*). They may not be able to take any decision and remain confused when exposed to a situation where they have to judge and pick one out of two choices (*ambivalence*). They lack self-care and often behave in appropriately in social situations because of poor cognitive functioning.

Their *mood/affect* is also variable and they may range from anxiety, fearfulness, distress and depression to anger outbursts. They may lose the ability to appreciate that they have a problem (*anosognosia or lack of insight*). They are usually more focused on the internal stimuli and thus keep smiling or laughing without any reason. They may act on their delusions and can sometimes turn *aggressive*. *However, premeditated violence by these patients is extremely uncommon.*

Symptoms must interfere with personal, social and occupational functioning. However, all kinds of psychotic disorders differ from each other with respect to the duration of disease and symptom profile as depicted in Table 3.2.2.

NEUROBIOLOGY

Before we discuss about schizophrenia, you must be aware of two major neurotransmitter systems in the brain: dopaminergic and glutaminergic (Fig. 3.2.2). We have four major dopaminergic pathways in the brain: mesocortical (1 in Fig. 3.2.2), mesolimbic (2 in Fig. 3.2.2) nigrao-striatal (3 in Fig. 3.2.2) and tuber-infundibular (not shown). Whereas the former two pathways are important for the symptomatology of schizophrenia, the latter two pathways explain the extrapyramidal symptoms and hyperprolectinaemia seen in patients on antipsychotics, respectively. These ascending pathways secrete dopamine that binds to presynaptic and postsynaptic D2 receptors and activate the neurons. These are termed as bottom-up pathways. D2 density is high in striatum and nucleus accumbens, whereas it is low in prefrontal cortex.

Glutamate system has seven pathways that originate in the cortex. Most important are cortico-cortical pathways—direct pathways stimulate neighbouring neurons (4 in Fig. 3.2.2), whereas the indirect pathway has intervening GABA neurons; thus, it inhibits the activity of neighbouring neurons (5 in Fig. 3.2.2). These neurons then project to the other brain areas forming other top-down pathways that include corticostriatal pathway (6 in Fig. 3.2.2), corticothalamic pathway (7 in Fig. 3.2.2), thalamocortical pathway (7 in Fig. 3.2.2), corticobrainstem pathway (8 in Fig. 3.2.2) and hippocampo–accumbens pathway (9 in Fig. 3.2.2). These top-down pathways modulate the functioning of bottom-up dopaminergic and other monoamine pathways (Fig. 3.2.2).

Schizophrenia spectrum disorders are caused by aberrant neurotransmission in the cortex. These patients are born with faulty NMDA receptors on the GABAergic interneurons in the indirect cortico-cortical pathway (5 in Fig. 3.2.2). Thus, there is a dysconnectivity between glutamate and GABA neuron leading to hypoactive GABA neuron. It translates to lesser inhibition of surrounding glutaminergic neurons. In other words, we can say that they remain hyperfunctional and release excessive glutamate

Table 3.2.2 Comparison of Schizophrenia Spectrum Disorders (DSM-5)

	Schizotypal Disorder	Brief Psychotic Disorder	Schizo Phreniform Disorder	Schizophrenia	Schizoaffective Disorder	Delusional Disorder
Age of onset	Adolescence	Adolescence or early adulthood	Late teens and mid thirties	Late teens and mid thirties	Early adulthood	More prevalent in elderly
Duration of symptoms	Life long	>1 day but <1 month	>1 month but <6 months	At least 6 months including prodrome and residual symptoms	Not specified	At least 1 month
Symptom profile	Ideas of reference Magical thinking Odd perceptual experiences Odd thinking and speech Paranoid ideas Inappropriate affect Eccentric behaviour Social anxiety	One or more of the following: Delusions Hallucinations Speech disturbances Disorganized behaviour	Two or more of the following: Delusions Hallucinations Speech disturbances Disorganized behaviour Negative symptoms	Two or more of the following: Delusions Hallucinations Speech disturbances Disorganized behaviour Negative symptoms	All of the following: 1. Major mood episode present with symptoms of schizophrenia 2. Delusions or hallucinations must be seen without mood symptoms any time during lifetime lasting at least 2 weeks 3. Most of the period of illness should have mood symptoms	One or more delusions is present Hallucinations are not present and if present, have delusional theme Disorganized behaviour not seen
Interfere with functioning	Present	Not necessary	Not necessary	Necessary	Not necessary	Except for the impact of delusion, function normal
Course	Stable course	Complete remission of symptoms	NA	Gradual progression; usually runs a chronic course with relapsing remitting pattern	Prognosis better than schizophrenia but worse than mood disorders	Some patients develop schizophrenia
Prevalence (United States)	3.9%	9%; more common in females	NA	0.3–0.7% (lifetime)	0.3% (lifetime); More common in females	0.2% (lifetime)

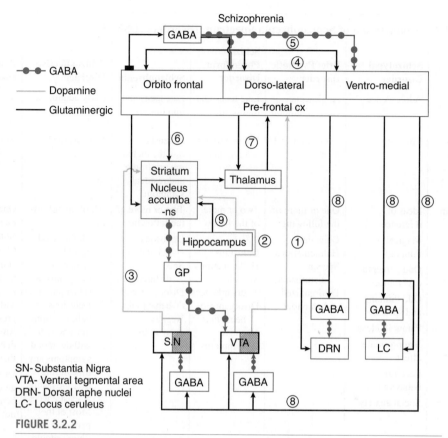

FIGURE 3.2.2

Neuronal pathways leading to schizophrenia spectrum disorders.

on the postsynaptic neurons (bottom-up neurons and other pathways), in turn, increasing their activity. As can be seen in Fig. 3.2.2, it leads to increased dopamine in nucleus accumbens (dopaminergic mesolimbic pathway; 2 in Fig. 3.2.2) and produce positive symptoms, eg, hallucinations, delusions, aggression and violence. Same effect is noticed when the hippocampal glutamate neurons become overactive for the same reason (hypofunction of intervening GABA neurons). However, as can be seen in Fig. 3.2.2, mesocortical pathway has intermediate GABA neuron. Its increased activity translates into a reduction of dopamine in the prefrontal cortex, thus producing negative, affective and cognitive symptoms with hypofrontality seen in these patients. While discussing the neurobiology, we will emphasize on two major symptoms of psychosis—hallucinations and delusions.

Hallucinating patients (experiencing auditory hallucinations) have aberrant activity in the auditory (superior and middle temporal gyri) and language areas (Wernicke's area in temporo-parietal area and Broca's area in inferior frontal gyrus). Aberrant activity is also seen in the anterior cingulate gyrus (that provides the behavioural directive to produce speech) and dorsolateral prefrontal cortex (that provides the sense of voluntary versus involuntary). Increased activity in the auditory areas in the presence of hypofunctional dorsolateral prefrontal cortex provides a sense that 'voices'are not originating in the brain, rather they are out of the voluntary control (passivity) and coming from outside. Altered corticothalamocortical circuits also play a role in this mechanism.

Neurobiology of delusion is more interesting. Learning theories suggest that we need to focus our attention on the stimuli (any information from the environment or from within) while learning and if we find the stimulus interesting, we learn that. Thus, a memory or a belief is formed and it depends upon how much 'salience' is associated with that stimulus. More the salience, higher is the chance of forming a memory. This is why we are able to keep track of a movie even after single exposure, whereas it may take a lot of effort to remember a lesson from the textbook. Once a belief is formed, it influences our perception and actions; in other words, it decides what we think and how we react to a given situation and so on. This experience will also generate a belief and thus this cycle continues. These beliefs must be robust so as to prevent our impulsive reaction in any given circumstance, but at the same time pliable enough so that our responses do not become fixed.

In the earliest phase of delusion formation, salience to the irrelevant environmental stimuli increases and the world appears changed. Because of poor cognitive functioning, the patients start paying attention to these irrelevant stimuli. These novel experiences increase the learning and thus lead to belief formation, ie, prior beliefs get changed in light of new evidences, because they are pliable.

As we have discussed, glutamate-induced excitation of meso-limbic tract increases in these disorders (Fig. 3.2.2) and these patients have poor filtering of environmental stimuli due to cortico-thalamocortical abnormality. This increases the information reaching the prefrontal cortex and also increases the dopamine activity (noise) in response to almost all environmental stimuli, irrespective of whether they should be attended or not! Release of dopamine increases the 'salience' of this information and compels the person to attend to these stimuli. So the sufferer starts experiencing 'novelty'. It inhibits the ongoing behaviour and the person starts finding new explanations for the events.

Experience of this novel situation also activates the hippocampus to increase the ventral tegmental area (VTA) dopaminergic tone. The prefrontal cortex gets information that it was not expecting (as it is a novel information) and initiates new learning through cholinergic mechanism (not shown in Fig. 3.2.2). Thus, overactivity of VTA increases the salience of all environmental stimuli, and reduced capacity to filter the information provides the 'the information provides the 'bizarre' character to the delusion.

Normally, when the prefrontal cortex finds that some information reaching the brain is not worthy to pay attention to, it reduces the firing of VTA neurons through hebenula (not shown in Fig. 3.2.2). This inhibition reverses the learning and promotes extinction (unlearning). However, this pathway is also deficient in psychosis and this is why the patients with delusions often hold the belief firmly, despite presented with contradictory evidences.

EPIDEMIOLOGY AND RISK FACTORS

Lifetime prevalence of schizophrenia in the United States is 0.3–0.7%. It has been found that late winters/early spring season may be a risk factor for schizophrenia; however, those born during summers are at higher risk for deficit form of schizophrenia (with prominent negative symptoms). Pregnancy and birth complication increase the risk, in addition to the genetic factors.

DIFFERENCES BETWEEN DSM-5 AND ICD-10 SYMPTOMATOLOGY

ICD-10 differs from the DSM-5 in certain symptomatology. However, as undergraduate, you may need to just understand the differences, rather than cramming them (Table 3.2.3).

Table 3.2.3 Differences in the ICD-10 from DSM-5

Schizotypal Disorder	Acute and Transient Psychotic Disorder	Schizophrenia	Induced Delusional Disorder	Schizoaffective Disorder	Persistent Delusional Disorder
Any four of the following symptoms: cold affect, odd behaviour, social withdrawal, magical thinking, panned ideas, rumination, illusions, odd thinking and quasi-psychotic episodes present for most of the time for at least 2 years.	Acute onset delusions, hallucinations and/or incoherent speech, with clear consciousness which reach to maximum intensity within 2 weeks. If symptoms match that of schizophrenia, they must remit within 1 month. If delusions are prominent and stable, it should be cleared within 3 months. If symptoms do not match that of schizophrenia, they should remit within 3 months	At least one of the following: (1) thought echo/thought broadcasting/thought withdrawal/thought insertion; (2) delusion of control; (3) third person or running commentary hallucinations; (4) bizarre delusions. Or at least two of the following: (1) persistent hallucinations in any modality with fleeting delusions; (2) incoherent speech, neologism; (3) catatonic behaviour; (4) negative symptoms are present for more than 1 month. It also categorizes it into various subtypes, eg, paranoid, hebephrenic, catatonic, undifferentiated, simple, residual and post-schizophrenic depression.	A person develops the same delusions when he/she comes into contact with a person who is already harbouring the delusion. This is also been described as shared delusions (Cotardsyndrome).	Disorders meet criteria for one of the mood disorders. Symptoms of schizophrenia must be present for at least 2 weeks. Symptoms of both the disorders must be present together for at least some part of the episode.	Person has nonbizzare delusion for at least 3 months in the absence of symptoms of schizophrenia.

DIFFERENTIAL DIAGNOSIS

Schizophrenia should be differentiated from all the disorders as mentioned in Table 3.2.2.

It must be differentiated from mood disorders. In mood disorders, the prominent complaints revolve around mood and it may be sad or euphoric. If psychotic features are seen in these conditions, they usually appear after prominent mood symptoms.

Flashbacks in the post-traumatic stress disorder (PTSD) may be mistaken for hallucinations. These can be differentiated on the basis of consistency of the content (flashbacks usually have same content) and history of major stress before the onset of symptoms.

DIAGNOSTIC FALLACIES

Paranoid ideas are not uncommon in obsessive–compulsive disorder. However, in this condition, ideas are intrusive, ego-dystonic and recurrent.

In case of improper information gathering, cluster A personality disorders, paranoid, schizoid and schizotypal personality disorders, may be mistaken for schizophrenia.

Delirium is often misdiagnosed as brief psychotic disorder, especially because of the presence of delusions and hallucinations. However, delirium is characterized by clouded consciousness, whereas it is clear in schizophrenia spectrum disorders.

Imagery can be misinterpreted for hallucinations, especially if the clinician does not enquire about all the characteristics of hallucinations (please refer to Chapter 1.2 on mental status examination).

Before mentioning the delusion, the clinician must spend adequate time with the patient and present all contradictory evidences and try to break it. If this is not done, an idea may be mistaken for delusion.

Wernicke's aphasia may be mistaken for loosening of association or incoherence.

MANAGEMENT

Both pharmacological and nonpharmacological therapies are used during the management of a patient with schizophrenia. Whereas symptoms are amenable only to the pharmacotherapy, nonpharmacological therapies are used during the rehabilitation process.

Most of the patients are not agitated and they may be managed on the outpatient basis. For schizophrenia and other psychotic disorders, antipsychotics are the mainstay of therapy. Two types of antipsychotics are available—first-generation and second-generation antipsychotics. These are available in oral as well as long-acting formulation. In general, oral medications are preferred; however, in noncompliant patients, long-acting injectable preparation may be preferred. In noncompliant patients, where injectable preparations are contraindicated, oral long-acting antipsychotic penfluridol may be used (Table 3.2.4).

Rarely, patients may be agitated and in this situation the main focus is to control the agitation. This can be achieved by physical restrain, using antipsychotics with hypnotic potential (haloperidol, chlorpromazine, olanzapine and qutiapine) or benzodiazepines (lorazepam and diazepam) or sedating antihistaminics (promethazine) or a combination of them. In noncooperative patients, injectable forms may be used. If aggression cannot be controlled, modified electroconvulsive therapy may be used. Behavioural therapy, eg, social skills training, may be used to rehabilitate the patients back in the society.

COURSE AND PROGNOSIS

Schizophrenia often runs a chronic course with relapsing–remitting pattern. In the early phase, positive symptoms predominate; however, as the disease progresses, dopamine neurotransmission lessen and negative symptoms appear. However, with the availability of antipsychotics, especially the atypical antipsychotics, the prognosis has improved. Many of these patients are able to lead a productive life, provided they remain adherent to the treatment.

These patients have higher chances of developing substance abuse, obsessive–compulsive disorder and panic disorder. These patients have higher rates of medical disorders, eg, weight gain, diabetes, metabolic syndrome owing to poor health behaviour and adverse effects of psychotropic drugs.

Table 3.2.4 Commonly used Antipsychotics in Treatment of Psychotic Spectrum Disorders

Name of the Drug	Preparation	Dose Range	Major Adverse Effects
First-generation antipsychotics			
Haloperidol	Oral	1–100 mg/day	Neuroleptic malignant syndrome (NMS), Extrapyramidal syndrome (EPS)
	Injectable	1–100mg/day	
	Long acting	40–80 mg every 2–4 weeks	
Trifluperazine	Oral	5–40 mg/day	EPS
Fluphenazine	Oral	1–40 mg/day	Agranulocytosis
	Long acting	25 mg every 1–4 weeks	Photosensitivity
Penfluperidol	Oral	10–40 mg once a week	EPS
Zuclopenthixol	Injectable, short-acting	50–150 mg every third day	EPS
	Injectable, long-acting	150–300 mg every 4 weeks	
Second-generation antipsychotics			
Clozapine	Oral	300–900 mg/day	NMS, seizures, agranulocytosis, EPS
Olanzepine	Oral	5–20 mg/day	Metabolic syndrome, sedation, weight gain, EPS
	Injectable	2.5–10 mg/day	
	Long-acting injectable	210–405 mg every 2 weeks (titrated to oral olanzapine doses)	
Paliperidone	Oral	3–12 mg/day	EPS
	Long-acting injectable	39–234 mg/month (titrated to oral paliperidone doses)	
Quetiapine	Oral	150–800 mg/day	Weight gain, NMS
Risperidone	Oral	2–12 mg/day	Weight gain, NMS, EPS
	Long acting injectable	25–50 mg every 2 weeks	
Ziprasidone	Oral	20–160 mg/day	Weight gain, NMS, EPS
Amisulpiride	Oral	400–800 mg/day	Hyperprolactinaemia

SUMMARY

- Schizophrenia and psychotic disorders can be seen as neurodevelopmental disorders.
- As per our present understanding, dysconnectivity of glutamate cells in prefrontal cortex is responsible for symptoms.
- These disorders present with delusions or hallucinations.
- Currently antipsychotics are the treatment of choice for these disorders.
- Untreated disorders lead to poor functioning, impart financial burden and adds to the burden of care on the family.

FURTHER READING

1. American Psychiatric Association. (2013). "Diagnostic and Statistical Manual of Mental Disorders." 5th edit, Author, Washington, DC.
2. Boksa P. (2009). On the Neurobiology of Hallucinations. *Journal of Psychiatry & Neuroscience*, 34:260–262.
3. Corlett P. R., Taylor J. R., Wang X. J., Fletcher P. C., and Krystal J. H. (2010). Toward a Neurobiology of Delusions. *Progress in Neurobiology*, 92:345–369.
4. World Health Organization. (1992). "The ICD-10 Classification of Mental and Behavioural Disorders: Clinical Descriptions and Diagnostic Guidelines." Author, Geneva.

ANXIETY DISORDERS

3.3

Ravi Gupta

Anxiety disorders are those disorders where anxiety is the prominent underlying symptom besides other clinical features. Anxiety is a common phenomenon and we all experience anxiety at times. It is usually associated with stress and, if you see Fig. 3.6.2, stress is not always bad. Thus, some amount of anxiety is important to keep you working towards a deadline. However, in certain conditions, it becomes pathological and starts interfering with performance. So, anxiety disorders are those clinical conditions where anxiety is the main symptom that keeps you away from performing your daily responsibilities. In this chapter, we will discuss about them.

NOSOLOGY

Nomenclature of anxiety disorders is more or less comparable between DSM-5 and ICD-10 (Table 3.3.1).

VIGNETTE

A 30-year-old man comes to you with complaints of feeling anxious and worrying over trivial issues. He says that he can feel his heart pounding most of the time and is not able to perform his job properly for the past 1 year because of these symptoms. At times, he develops intense anxiety that is beyond his control, with palpitations, tremors and sweating that last for approximately 15–20 min. During this period, he feels weak as if his legs would give way. On further questioning, it appeared that these symptoms develop when he has to make a presentation in front of the board members. He is a banker and thus he has to make presentations frequently and meet people from all strata of the group. He also feels nervous when he has to go to a public meeting because he feels that everybody is staring at him and judging him. During these times, it often comes to his mind that he is improperly dressed and people would make fun of him. He is not able to have his meals in such circumstances because he feels that he would not be eating properly. Physical examination was within normal limits. Examination of his mental status revealed anxiety during specific situations. Based on the history and examination, diagnosis of specific phobia was made.

CLINICAL FEATURES

A basic complaint of such patients is the feeling of anxiety. This anxiety can be of low grade that remains all the time or can be intense but short lasting. They often complain of symptoms that suggest sympathetic arousal, eg, heightened alertness, feeling anxious, nervousness, tremulousness, palpitations, high pulse rate, frequent urination, sweaty palms and soles and generalized weakness.

Table 3.3.1 Comparative Nosology of Anxiety Disorders

DSM-5	ICD-10
Specific phobia	Specific isolated phobias
Social anxiety disorder/social phobia	Social phobia
Panic Disorder	Panic disorder
Agoraphobia	Agoraphobia
Generalized anxiety disorder	Generalized anxiety disorder

Some of the disorders, eg, phobias, have anxiety that appears in specific situations. Not only the actual exposure but merely the thought of being in that situation may provoke the anxiety. Some commonly reported situations are social gathering, seeing blood, performing on the stage, going out of the house alone and in closed spaces. These patients try to avoid such situations. Termination of exposure to the situation/stimulus ends anxiety.

In generalized anxiety disorder, anxiety remains all the time and the main part is worry. Somatic symptoms are also present but they are less intense. Many of these patients also complain of poor-quality sleep or difficulty in falling asleep. Contrary to generalized anxiety disorder, panic disorder is an episodic illness that may start for no apparent reason and lasts for approximately 15–20 min. It is characterized by intense anxiety, with palpitations, tremulousness, appearance of weakness and sweating.

Symptoms must interfere with social, personal or occupational functioning of the patient (Table 3.3.2).

NEUROBIOLOGY

These disorders present with two core symptoms–first, symptoms that suggest fear, eg, panic or phobia and, second, worrying. Thus, these disorders involve two circuits of the brain; fear is regulated by amygdala-centred circuits and worry by cortico–striato–thalamo–cortical (CSTC) loops. First, we will talk about fear; fear is an emotion that leads to sympathetic arousal. This arousal manifests as a change in motor activity and vital parameters; in addition, it leads to an increase in cortisol. We have earlier discussed that fear is evoked not only on exposure to the stimulus but also with the thought of having the same experience again. These observations suggest that the seat of fear, the amygdala, has to have connections with emotional areas of prefrontal cortex, locus ceruleus, periaquductal grey and brainstem nuclei that control vital activity, eg, breathing, heart rate, hypothalamus and hippocampus (Fig. 10.1.4). Similarly, worrying requires activity in the CSTC loops, details of which are yet to be elucidated. This is the general understanding of symptoms in anxiety disorders.

When we go for a more specific neurobiological mechanism, we need to understand the disorders with reference to a network model.

Cingulo-opercular network (CON) is responsible for detecting errors or conflicts. This is also known as salience network and is responsible for appreciating negative responses like negative emotions and pain. This network is highly active among patients with anxiety disorders making them more sensitive

Table 3.3.2 Symptomatology of different Anxiety Disorders

	Specific Phobias	Social Phobia	Agoraphobia	Panic Disorder	Generalized Anxiety Disorder
Stimulus	Very specific, eg, seeing animals, height, water, blood and closed spaces	Situations where a person may be scrutinized by others eg, talking to people, delivering speech	Present;symptoms usually appear while using public transport, open spaces, closed spaces, crowd or going alone outside	May be present or may not be present	Not present
Consistency	Exposure of this environment always evoke anxiety	Exposure of this environment always evoke anxiety	Exposure of this environment always evoke anxiety	Persistent worry that they would develop similar attacks	Not applicable
Anticipation	Present that they would develop symptoms in such situations	Present that they would develop symptoms in such situations	Present that they would develop symptoms in such situations	May be present	Not applicable
Rationale	Perceived anxiety is out of proportion	Perceived anxiety is out of proportion	Perceived anxiety is out of proportion	–	Not applicable
Avoidance	Always try to avoid such situations	Always try to avoid such situations	Always try to avoid such situations	Always try to avoid situations that may provoke panic attack	Not applicable
Duration	At least 6 months	At least 6 months	At least 6 months	At least 1 month	At least 6 months
Other symptoms		Feel that they would be negatively evaluated by people	Feel that they would not be able to escape in case they develop anxiety or that they will not get immediate help if they would develop panic-like symptoms or any other symptoms that would make them incapacitated, eg, if they would fall down	Intense anxiety episodes lasting few minutes associated with somatic symptoms of sympathetic arousal	Consistent worry and anxiety about a variety of situations: whether I would be able to perform well, what would happen to my family, which are beyond the control of the patient and associated with somatic symptoms, eg, fatigue, poor concentration, muscle tension, irritable mood

towards negative or apparently negative stimuli. It also detects behavioural errors so as to modify the cognitive strategies according to the context.

Second is the fronto-parietal network (FPN) or executive control network. As the name suggests, this network helps in changing the strategies in the conflicting situations. This network responds back to CON to adjust CON's activity in judging the stimuli. This network is also in connection with the amygdala to control its output (top-down control). In these patients, the connectivity between these two networks is disturbed. That is why anxious patients perceive nonthreatening stimulus as threatening. Moreover, poor top-down control adds to the appearance of sympathetic symptoms, as mentioned above.

Third, ventral attention network (VAN) helps us to focus our attention on a given stimulus. Anxiety disorder patients have a high activity in this region that brings and maintains their attention to even a nonemotional stimulus. This network also has connection with amygdala and, in patients with anxiety disorders, this connection is strong. This, in part, suggests why these patients have high anxiety on sudden appearance of a stimulus.

Fourth is the default mode network (DMN) that is important for emotional regulation, cognitive control over emotions (regulation of emotion with rationale thoughts) and extinction of fear with repeated presentation of fearful stimulus. It has decreased activity in patients with anxiety disorders and its connection with amygdala is also weak. This is why patients with anxiety disorders, even after knowing that the stimulus is nonthreatening, become and remain anxious (Fig. 3.3.1).

EPIDEMIOLOGY AND RISK FACTORS

Prevalence of specific phobia in the United States is approximately 7–9%; 7% for social phobia and 3% for panic disorder. Agoraphobia is usually seen in 1–2% and similar rates have been reported for generalized anxiety disorder. Prevalence of anxiety disorders is lower in Asians. In general, their prevalence increases from childhood to adolescence but reduces thereafter with advancing age. Women have higher prevalence than men. Specific phobia usually appears after experiencing a trauma in a specific situation or by others' experiences of trauma in that particular situation.

Differences in the diagnostic criteria of anxiety disorders between ICD-10 from DSM-5 are summarized in Table 3.3.3.

DIFFERENTIAL DIAGNOSIS

These disorders must be differentiated from each other. They must be differentiated from symptoms that may emerge with other medical conditions, eg, bronchial asthma, pheochromocytoma, hyperthyroidism or with the use of drugs, eg, sympathomimetic drugs. All these conditions may induce symptoms of anxiety disorders.

They must be differentiated from symptoms occurring during intoxication or withdrawal of substance of abuse suggested by history, clinical examination and screening for drugs of abuse.

Some people are shy because of their nature. This should be differentiated from social phobia. This must also be differentiated from autistic spectrum disorder (ASD), cluster A and cluster C personality disorders and psychotic disorders with the help of age of onset of symptoms (childhood in ASD;

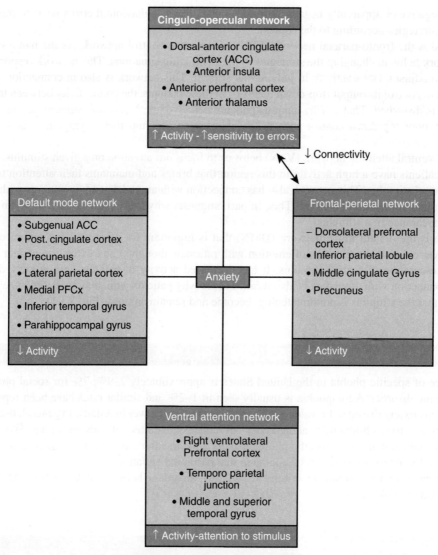

FIGURE 3.3.1

Functional neurobiology of anxiety disorders.

adolescence in personality disorders) and associated symptoms (hallucinations and delusions in psychosis; stereotypy in ASD).

Specific phobias must be differentiated from obsessive–compulsive disorder (OCD), eg, a person having obsessions regarding contamination may try to avoid socialization. However, in OCD, main focus will be the contamination rather than the feeling of being criticized.

Table 3.3.3 Difference in ICD-10 from DSM-5

Specific Phobias	Social Phobia	Agoraphobia	Panic Disorder	Generalized Anxiety Disorder
Includes situations like closed spaces	–	Does not include situations like public transport and closed spaces	–	–
No duration criteria, one episode is enough	No duration criteria, one episode is enough	No duration criteria, one episode is enough	No duration criteria	–
Associated symptoms, eg, sympathetic arousal, chest and abdominal symptoms, mental symptoms, must be present	Associated symptoms, eg, sympathetic arousal, chest and abdominal symptoms, mental symptoms, must be present	Associated symptoms, eg, sympathetic arousal, chest and abdominal symptoms, mental symptoms, must be present	Associated symptoms, eg, sympathetic arousal, chest and abdominal symptoms, mental symptoms, must be present	Associated symptoms, eg, sympathetic arousal, chest and abdominal symptoms, mental symptoms, must be present

DIAGNOSTIC FALLACIES

Social phobia may be mistaken for the delusion of reference or other way round. Thus, a careful questioning is required to reach to a diagnosis.

Many of the symptoms of depression overlap with generalized anxiety disorder, at least superficially. Thus, a careful questioning is required to ascertain a diagnosis.

MANAGEMENT

Two kinds of therapies are available for the management of these disorders—pharmacological and behavioural. Among the pharmacological therapies, benzodiazepines are used to control acute attack of anxiety and for the short-term treatment of anxiety. It is better to use long-acting benzodiazepines (eg, clonazepam 0.25–2 mg/day; diazepam 2–10 mg/day) as they require less-frequent dosage. Selective serotonin reuptake inhibitors (escitalopram 5–20 mg/day; sertraline 25–100 mg/day; paroxetine 12.5–37.5 mg/day) can also control anxiety by acting on 5-HT1A receptors. However, they take around 2–3 weeks to show their effect. Dictum for their use is to start low and go slow, especially in these cases, owing to their anxiogenic potential.

Behavioural therapies include relaxation techniques, systemic desensitization and exposure and response prevention. For details, please refer to Chapter 9.1.

COURSE AND PROGNOSIS

These are the disorders that have relapsing and remitting course in most of the patients; however, others may experience complete remission after treatment of one episode.

SUMMARY

- Anxiety disorders are common and reduce in prevalence as we age.
- These disorders result from decreased activity in neural networks that control the emotions and executive functions.
- There is increased activity in neural networks that provoke anxiety.
- These disorders can be effectively managed by therapy.
- Behavioural therapies are an important aspect of management of these disorders.

FURTHER READING

1. American Psychiatric Association. (2013). "Diagnostic and Statistical Manual of Mental Disorders." 5th edit, Author, Washington, DC.
2. Sylvester C. M., Corbetta M., Raichle M.E., et al. (2012). Functional Network Dysfunction in Anxiety and Anxiety Disorders. *Trends in Neurosciences*, 35:527–535.
3. World Health Organization. (1992). "The ICD-10 Classification of Mental and Behavioural Disorders: Clinical Descriptions and Diagnostic Guidelines." Author, Geneva.

OBSESSIVE–COMPULSIVE AND RELATED DISORDERS

3.4

Ravi Gupta

'Obsessive–compulsive and related disorders' is a category of disorders where the main feature is recurrent thoughts, impulse or images that intrude a person's mind/consciousness against his/her will (obsessions). These obsessions are often, but not always, accompanied by some kinds of mental or physical acts (compulsions) that a person has to accomplish to compensate the obsessions.

This category includes a number of disorders, eg, obsessive–compulsive disorder (OCD), body dysmorphic disorder, hoarding disorder, trichotillomania, excoriation (skin picking) and, lastly, substance use disorder.

In these disorders, recurring thoughts compel a person to act upon it, and if not acted upon, lead to significant amount of anxiety. This is one reason why in the earlier classification (DSM-IV-TR), OCD was kept in the category of anxiety disorders. Similarly, body dysmorphic disorder was kept in the category of somatic symptoms disorders and trichotillomania was recognized as an impulse control disorder in DSM-IV-TR. Although, substance use disorder share the neurobiology with these disorders, however, because of the use of a specific substance, their specific effect on the organ systems, and having a different modality for the treatment, it is considered as a separate group of disorder.

NOSOLOGY

There is a difference in the nomenclature of these disorders between DSM-5 and ICD-10 (Table 3.4.1).

Table 3.4.1 Comparative Nosology of OCD and Spectrum Disorders	
DSM-5	**ICD-10**
OCD	OCD
Body dysmorphic disorder	–
Hoarding disorder	–
Trichotillomania	–
Excoriation	–

VIGNETTE

A 27-year-old woman presented with complaints of repeated hand washing. Her husband complained that she washes her hands every 2–3 h to the extent that the skin of her hands has been damaged. She also does not let him or any of the other family members touch the utensils unless they wash their hands to her satisfaction. She does not allow them to bring the footwear inside the house and if they do so, she would mop the whole house, leaving behind other urgent works in hand. When she was interviewed separately, she said that she does not get satisfaction that her hands are clean enough after washing them for once. A thought that her hands are still untidy keeps haunting her and she is not able to get rid of it, unless she washes them many times. She further mentioned that she knows what she was doing was wrong, but cannot get rid of the thought. Whenever somebody touches the utensils, she feels that they have gone dirty and she compels the family to wash their hands before touching anything, otherwise she would wash the utensils using a detergent. She agrees that her preoccupation with cleanliness is excessive, unrealistic and she should not do it. However, she mentions that she has recurrent thoughts regarding cleanliness and to get rid of the thoughts she has to follow these acts. General physical examination did not contribute to the diagnosis. Examination of mental status disclosed anxiety and obsessions and compulsions that were ego dystonic. Based on the history and examination, diagnosis of OCD was made.

CLINICAL PICTURE

OCD can present in a variety of forms; contamination, counting, checking and symmetry are the common presentations. Patients with contamination type are fearful of catching an infection or getting dirty. They have these obsessions and to control these obsessions, they remain engaged in some rituals, eg, repeatedly washing their hands or repetitive cleaning the house or objects. Counting type of OCD presents with recurrent counting before they proceed to next step in any work. This counting may include counting currency notes or steps. Checking type OCD presents with repeated checking for the gas knob, locks, door bolts and they are not able to satisfy themselves unless they do it several times. People with symmetry type of symptoms prefer to keep things arranged in a symmetrical manner. If somebody disturbs the symmetry, they become anxious and irritable. Some people may have sexual thoughts/images or paranoid thoughts as obsessions. These thoughts/images/urges and acts are ego dystonic at least during some part of the symptomatic period, ie, these patients become perturbed of these symptoms.

Patients with body dysmorphic disorder feel that some part of their body is improper or not in shape, and to compensate for these thoughts, they keep on checking the same part again and again.

Hoarding disorder is manifested by difficulty in discarding the objects that do not have any emotional or monitory value or even when their usefulness cease to exist. They become distressed when somebody asks them to part away from the junk and they keep on collecting old clothes, utensils, objects, books, papers, etc., without using them for long durations.

Repeated pulling of hair and picking of skin characterize trichotillomania and excoriation, respectively. These people often try to prevent themselves from doing these acts, but they fail to do so because of the mounting tension. The term 'mounting anxiety' depicts a state of gradually increasing anxiety till the person acts on the urge. They spend a significant amount of time in these activities and become

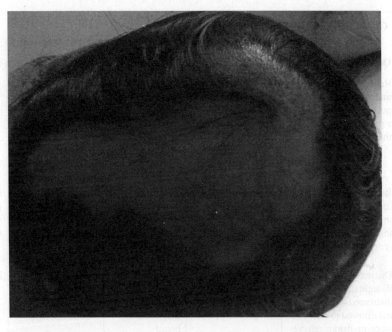

FIGURE 3.4.1

Scalp of a person with tricotillomania.

(Source: *Himalayan Hospital, Dehradun*).

distressed. Most commonly affected areas are those which are easily accessible to hand, eg, scalp (Fig. 3.4.1), face, chest, abdomen and limbs.

Although these disorders share a common pathophysiological link, still they differ in clinical presentation (Table 3.4.2).

NEUROBIOLOGY

Neurobiology of the OCD and related disorders involve abnormality in the cortico–striato–thalamo–cortical (CSTC) circuit (Fig. 3.4.2). Structural neuroimaging has shown a change in volume of orbitofrontal cortex, anterior cingulate cortex, caudate nucleus and thalamus. It is considered that an imbalance between the direct and indirect CSTC circuits (OCD loop) that originate from the orbitofrontal cortex leads to the increased information exchange between the thalamus and orbitofrontal cortex. Both of these areas have been found hyperactive in OCD patients in functional neuroimaging. However, OCD is associated with a negative change in cognitive functioning, ie, these patients may not be able to inhibit the hyperactivity of thalamus and orbitofrontal cortex using their 'thinking brain'. Consistent with this clinical information, brain areas that are important for the cognitive functioning, ie, thinking and decision making, eg, dorsolateral prefrontal cortex,

Table 3.4.2 Comparison of Disorders

	OCD	Body Dysmorphic Disorder	Hoarding Disorder	Trichotillomania	Excoriation (Skin Picking)
Thoughts	Recurrent intrusive and undesired thoughts, impulse and images where a person tries to ignore them (obsessions)	Always preoccupied that some part of their body is does not appear good	Individual perceive that they need to save the item even after its importance ceases to exist without any actual utility	–	–
Acts	Repetitive physical or mental acts, eg, washing, checking or praying, repeating words (compulsions)	Repetitive checking in mirror or compare their body parts with that of others	Storing the items to the extent that the house become overfilled with them	Repeated hair pulling along with attempts to reduce it	Repeated hair pulling along with attempts to reduce it
Distress	Distressed with thoughts;also feel distressed if they are not allowed to do so;compulsions relieve the anxiety	Distress present because of the preoccupation	When they are asked to discard the items that they want to hoard	Present	Present
Time spent	At least 1 h per day	Not specified	Not specified	Not specified	Not specified
Duration	Not specified	Not specified	Not specified	Not specified	Not specified

anterior cingulate gyrus and cerebellum (habit learning), have been found to have low activity in these patients.

It has been proposed that different symptoms of OCD are manifested by different neural systems. The emotional symptoms, eg, impulsiveness and anxiety that are associated with checking/counting are regulated by the anterior cingulate cortex and its connections with the striatum. On the other hand, contamination type of OCD requires somatic perception; hence, it involves connections between temporal lobe and ventrolateral prefrontal cortex. These areas are connected to the OCD loop through orbitofrontal cortex. The cognitive part of this type of OCD involves a dysfunction in the dorsolateral prefrontal cortex (Fig. 3.4.2).

EPIDEMIOLOGY AND RISK FACTORS

One-year prevalence of OCD is around 1.1% in the United States. Female gender is a risk factor. In the United States, body dysmorphic disorder is seen in 2.4% people with higher rates among the people who approach for various cosmetic surgeries, including oromaxillofacial surgery, orthodontic surgery and dermatology clinics. Prevalence of hoarding disorder is not known. Like other disorders of this group, trichotillomania and excoriation also affects 1–2% people with female preponderance.

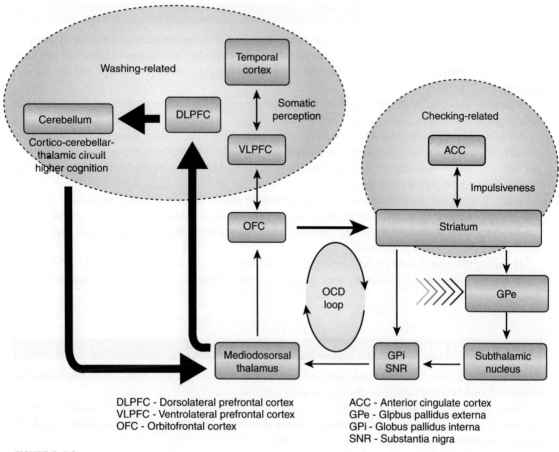

FIGURE 3.4.2

Neurobiology of OCD.

(Reproduced with permission from: *Nakao T, Okada K, Kanba S. Neurobiological model of obsessive–compulsive disorder: Evidence from recent neuropsychological and neuroimaging findings. Psychiatry ClinNeurosci 2014; 68: 587-605).*

DIFFERENCE BETWEEN DSM-5 AND ICD-10

ICD-10 differs from DSM-5 in certain aspects of diagnostic guidelines. This is presented in Table 3.4.3.

Table 3.4.3 Differences in ICD-10 from DSM-5

Obsessive–Compulsive Disorder	Body Dysmorphic Disorder	Hoarding Disorder	Trichotillomania	Excoriation
Specifies a duration of symptoms of at least 2 weeks	–	–	Requires 'an intense urge to pull their hair with a mounting tension that is relieved by the act'	–

DIFFERENTIAL DIAGNOSIS

These disorders must be differentiated from each other by the symptom profile. Obsessions must be differentiated from worries as seen in generalized anxiety disorder, and ruminations which are seen in depression. Unlike obsessions, worries and ruminations are not considered foreign and are not ego dystonic.

Compulsions must be differentiated from tics and stereotyped movements seen across a variety of conditions and disorders. These are not ego dystonic.

OCD must be differentiated from obsessive–compulsive (OC) personality disorder. OC personality disorder usually starts in adolescence and does not have the symptoms mentioned above. Rather, patients with OC personality disorder bear a rigidity regarding the rules, methods and symmetry to the extent of maladaptation to their environment.

Body dysmorphic disorder needs differentiation from illness anxiety disorder, delusional disorder and eating disorders. Primary focus in illness anxiety disorders is anxiety regarding having an illness, not the body part. Patients with eating disorder often have a body-image misperception and do not focus on a particular part of the body.

Hoarding disorder should be differentiated from accumulation of objects secondary to a delusion.

Trichotillomania and excoriation must be differentiated from factitious disorder and delusional disorder.

DIAGNOSTIC FALLACIES

Some amount of preoccupation with appearance is common among adolescents. They should not be diagnosed with body dysmorphic disorder in such circumstances.

Many people have repetitive thoughts; however, these thoughts are not considered as alien and they are able to shift their attention when desired. These should not be considered as obsessions. Similarly worries about day-to-day matters are not obsessions.

Hoarding disorders should not be diagnosed if the symptoms arise after any kind of brain trauma—accidental, infectious, stroke or iatrogenic (neurosurgery). Similarly, if the symptoms appear in settings of neurodevelopmental disorders (eg, autistic spectrum disorder, intellectual disability and Prader–Willi syndrome) or neurocognitive disorders, hoarding disorder should not be diagnosed.

Hair pulling and excoriation to improve the looks (eg, threading and removing pimples) should not be mistaken for the trichotillomania and excoriation.

MANAGEMENT

Mainstay of the therapy is pharmacological treatment. These disorders may be controlled by the use of selective serotonin reuptake inhibitors (eg, fluoxetine 20–80 mg/day; sertraline 50–200 mg/day) or tricyclics with relatively higher serotonin activity, eg, clomipramine (25–150 mg/day). Doses are often higher than those used in anxiety disorders and depressive disorders. To control the associated anxiety, benzodiazepines (eg, clonazepam 0.25–2 mg/day) may be used.

Nonpharmacological therapy is effective for OCD, especially when it is accompanied with pharmacological treatment. One of the therapy for OCD is exposure and response prevention (please refer to Chapter 9.1).

COURSE AND PROGNOSIS

These disorders usually start during adolescence and run a chronic course with multiple relapses unless adequately treated.

SUMMARY

- OCD and related disorders have in common the recurrent thoughts and/or ritualistic behaviour.
- Initiation of treatment at appropriate time can improve the clinical condition.
- Neurobiologically, it is related to abnormality in cortico–striato–thamalo–cortical loop.
- Serotonin reuptake inhibitors are effective in management of these disorders.

FURTHER READING

1. American Psychiatric Association. (2013). "Diagnostic and Statistical Manual of Mental disorders." 5th edit, Author, Washington, DC.
2. Nakao T., Okada K., and Kanba S. (2014). Neurobiological Model of Obsessive–Compulsive Disorder: Evidence From Recent Neuropsychological and Neuroimaging Findings. *Psychiatry and Clinical Neurosciences*, 68:587–605.
3. World Health Organization. (1992). "The ICD-10 Classification of Mental and Behavioural Disorders: Clinical Descriptions and Diagnostic Guidelines." Author, Geneva.

CULTURE-SPECIFIC DISORDERS

3.5

Ravi Gupta

Culture-specific disorders depict constellation of those behavioural symptoms that are deviant from normal behaviour since most of the people do not experience and manifest them. Some of them are regarded as normal by most of the people in that particular culture, but not in other cultures. Interestingly, unlike other psychiatric disorders, which have similar symptomatology across cultures, these presentations have limited geographical presentations and even in a given geographical area may be confined to a specific culture.

It is yet to be defined whether they should be regarded as 'disorders' but they are often the cause for the distress. It has been argued that these symptoms can be culture-specific presentation of a known psychiatric disorder and thus they deserve clinical attention. This culture-specific presentation can be explained by the learning theory—we all learn to express our emotions in a particular fashion by imitating our parents, friends and people around us and try to keep the manner of expression in that situation according to social or cultural norms. To substantiate this theory, it has been experimentally proved that even the six basic emotions–happiness, surprise, anger, fear, disgust and sadness–have different presentations across cultures and the way of presentation is usually learned.

Thus, the scientific world is still debating whether these culture-specific disorders should be considered psychiatric disorders. Moreover, owing to their limited geographical presentation, their neurobiology is not known. Thus, the issue is more complex than it appears. It is worthwhile to mention that DSM-5 does not list them; however, in ICD-10, they are listed in the Annexure 2.

Still, understanding of these disorders is important for you because you may encounter a number of patients with these disorders in your clinical practice. In this chapter, we will discuss the culture-specific disorders that are prevalent in India and will list some other culture-specific disorders that are seen in other parts of the world.

DHAT SYNDROME

This is a common culture-specific disorder, often seen among adolescent boys. It is also seen in China where it is known as Shen-kui. The adolescent often complains of losing some whitish discharge along with urine, which he considers as semen. In Indian culture, semen has been associated with vigour and is considered precious. Because of this reason, the patient remains excessively concerned with the loss of semen, feels fatigued throughout the day and loses appetite. The patient also complains about declining memory and physical performance.

This belief originates with the cultural knowledge of production of semen. Culturally, in India it is believed that 40 meals will generate one drop of blood; 40 drops of blood will generate one drop of marrow (majja) and, lastly, 40 drops of marrow (majja) will be required for the production of one drop of semen.

It may be considered as an equivalent to the somatic symptoms disorder.

KORO

It is seen in Eastern India. Affected individuals usually present with anxiety or panic along with the fear of retraction of genitalia in their body. It can be seen in both males and females, men will focus on their penis and females on their breasts and external genitalia—labia and vulva. It has an abrupt onset. Sufferer often worries that these symptoms will culminate into an end to his life. They provide a variety of responses that include grasping their genitalia themselves or asking a family member to do so. Some people may use splints and other devices to hold the genitalia from disappearing within the body. This may be equated to somatic symptoms disorder.

POSSESSION DISORDER

This is common in all parts of India. The symptoms usually start in an emotionally charged environment, eg, during a mass prayer, but may occur without it as well. The affected individual shows as if he/she is possessed by a spirit, which either can be of a God (*devi* or *devta*) or an evil spirit (ghost). They often ask other people to fulfil their demands as they are considered as a 'special' persons by the other people in community.

Often these patients are brought when this disorder start occurring outside the emotionally charged environment or when it starts occurring frequently. ICD-10 considers it as conversion disorder and it may be treated on similar lines.

ASCETIC SYNDROME

Professor N.N. Wig first described this in 1972 among adolescents and young adults who showed a change in behaviour and became socially withdrawn. They practiced sexual abstinence, lost the concerns for their physical appearance and engaged in religious practices.

SUCHI-BAI

It is seen in West Bengal, especially among the Hindu widows. They have a preoccupation for cleanliness and keep washing their hands, body, clothes and utensils for a long time. Some of them even remain immersed in river for a long time.

GILHARI SYNDROME

This was first reported in Western Rajasthan and is also known as lizard syndrome. Patients presented with a lump on their back that is mobile and believed to reach the throat finally, which would eventually lead to death.

Table 3.5.1 summarizes some culture-bound syndromes reported across various cultures.

DIFFERENTIAL DIAGNOSIS

Patients with Dhat syndrome may actually have discharge of prostatic fluid (which is colourless and of mucinous consistency, slightly more viscous than saliva) or calcium oxalate crystals in urine, which they mistake for semen. Thus, they should be investigated for urethritis, acute prostatitis and oxalate crystals in urine.

Weight gain is associated with increment of subcutaneous fat in the pelvic region (around genitalia) and in the abdomen, providing the misperception of genital retraction. Thus, obesity should be looked for in Koro.

All these short-lasting episodes must be differentiated from epilepsy.

MANAGEMENT

Patients with Dhat syndrome and Koro should be provided the knowledge regarding the anatomy and physiology of the reproductive system, which is related to their symptoms.

As we have already discussed, these disorders may indeed be the culture-specific presentation of other psychiatric disorders (somatic symptoms disorder, anxiety disorders and mood disorders). Thus, they may be managed on the lines of respective disorder.

Table 3.5.1 Culture Bound Syndromes Reported Across Various Cultures

Name	Geographical Area	Symptoms
Latah	Indonesia, Malayasia	This is seen during the trauma followed by involuntary echolalia, echopraxia and trans-like state. Can be considered a part of conversion disorder.
Nerfiza	Egypt, Central and South America, Mexico, Northern Europe	This is more common among women and characterized by anxiety, generalized body aches, sleep disturbances, nausea, vomiting and fatigue. Can be considered as depression.
Pe-leng	Southeast Asia and China	Patients present with anxiety and fear of cold winds that can lead to lethargy, loss of virility and, ultimately, death. Patients often wear excessive clothes to protect themselves.
Pibloktoq	Arctic area	Fatigue and sadness followed by seizure-like episodes. Patients may run into snow, tear their cloths and show echolalia and echopraxia. Episodes lasts for minutes and patients often do not have the memory of the same.

SUMMARY

- Culture-related disorders are limited to geographical boundaries.
- They may be culture-specific presentation of psychiatric disorders.

FURTHER READING

1. American Psychiatric Association. (2013). "Diagnostic and Statistical Manual of Mental Disorders." 5th edit, Author, Washington, DC.
2. Balhara Y. P. S. (2011). Culture-Bound Syndrome: Has it Found its Right Niche? *Indian Journal of Psychological Medicine*, 33:210–215.
3. Jack R. E., Garrod O. G. B, Yu H., Caldara R., and Schyns P. G. (2012). Facial Expressions of Emotion Are not Culturally Universal. *Proceedings of National Academy of Sciences*, 109:7241–7244.
4. Malhotra H. K., and Wig N. N. (1975). Dhat Syndrome: A Culture-Bound Sex Neurosis of the Orient. *Archives of Sexual Behavior*, 4:519–528.
5. Neki J. S. (1972). The Ascetic Syndrome (Mimeo). pp. 1–5. All Indian Institute of Medical Sciences, New Delhi India.
6. Verma K. K., Bhojak M. M., Singhal A. K., Jhirwal O. P., and Khunteta A. (2001). "Gilahari (Lizard) Syndrome" Is It a New Culture Bound Syndrome? - A Case Report. *Indian Journal of Psychiatry*, 43:70–72.
7. World Health Organization. (1992). "The ICD-10 Classification of Mental and Behavioural Disorders: Clinical Descriptions and Diagnostic Guidelines." Author, Geneva.

STRESS AND PSYCHIATRIC DISORDERS

Ravi Gupta

Stress is also known as tension and this can either be physical or emotional. In its simplest form, physical stress is experienced when somebody moves a part of his/her body beyond the normal limits, eg, stretching the arm or flexing the forearm forcefully. Resultant physical stress evokes pain and thus, in turn, induces emotional stress. Thus, all physical stresses are associated with negative emotions and conjure emotional stresses as well. Each of us has different capacity to bear physical stress that is determined by physical strength and flexibility.

On the other hand, emotional stress occurs in situations involving emotional conflicts, eg, when a person has to choose one option between the two or after receiving appalling information. Here, person may not feel any 'physical pain' but 'emotional pain' is experienced. Like physical stress, capacity to bear emotional stress also differs from person to person and depends upon the resilience of the neural network of the brain.

Brain is the main organ of the body that handles the stress and tries to reduce its brunt. In doing so, it initiates the sympathetic reaction along with activation of the hypothalamo–pituitary–adrenal (HPA) axis and prepares the body to counteract stress. Sometimes, and in some persons who have high resilience, this reaction produces protective effects but in those with low resilience, stress may injure the brain and the body. In this chapter, we will discuss about the neurobiology of stress and the disorders that are related to the stress.

NEUROBIOLOGY

As we have already discussed, the brain not only modulates reaction to the stress but also bears the consequences. Before we talk about stress pathways, we must know the pathways that process the information, which reaches the brain. It starts with sensing the stimuli from the environment or from inside the body through sensory organs and then it is transmitted to the respective association cortices. From the association cortex, this is then conveyed to the prefrontal cortex, which compares it with already stored information (ie, memories) and assess its significance. Finally, a decision is taken after analysing the stimulus from multiple aspects and, if the situation appears stressful, the stress response is recruited. Thus, the problem is perceived (consciously recognized) and this can evoke the typical stress response by recruiting 'stress-related pathways' which leads to multiple consequences (Fig. 3.6.1). Depending upon the duration, stress can be divided into two types: acute and chronic.

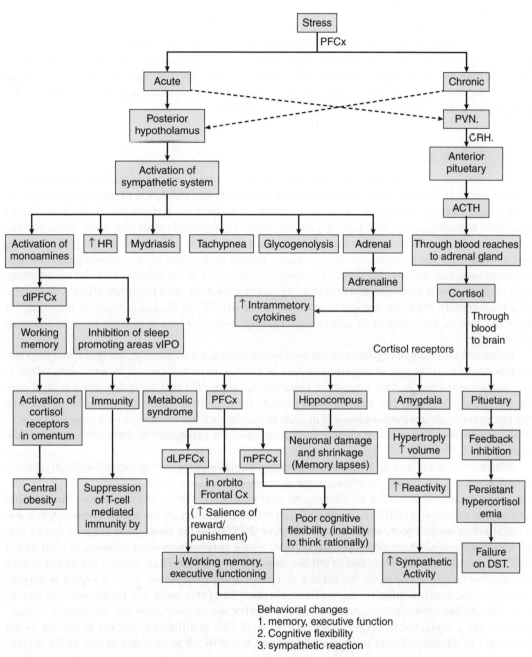

FIGURE 3.6.1

Neurobiology of stress. Dashed line show minor contribution. PVN, paraventricular nucleus; ACTH, adrenocorticotrophic hormone; HR, heart rate; PFCx, prefrontal cortex; dlPFCx, dorsolateral prefrontal cortex; mPFCx, medial prefrontal cortex; vlPO, ventrolateral preoptic area; DST, dexamethasone suppression test.

ACUTE STRESS

Sympathetic system plays an important role during acute stress so as to prepare us for 'fight or flight'. Acute stress usually lasts for few minutes to few hours, whereas chronic stress denotes any stress lasting more than few hours, though the differentiation is arbitrary. You can appreciate the consequences of acute and chronic stress in Fig. 3.6.1. Acute stress is a common and unavoidable experience and it appears that it does not produce long-lasting harmful effects.

CHRONIC STRESS

On the other hand, a plethora of literature suggests that chronic stress has multiple deleterious effects on the body, which may be extended to, but not limited to, modulation of immune system (both cellular and humoral immunity), adverse metabolic consequences and ultimately predisposing an individual to multiple disorders. Contrary to activation of sympathetic system in acute stress, chronic stress exerts its effects through cortisol (Fig. 3.6.1). It mediates its effect through the glucocorticoid and mineralocorticoid receptors on various organs. During stress, there is an increased glutamate neurotransmission that destroys the neurons leading to dysfunction of the affected area. It also interferes with the long-term potentiation and thus memory lapses appear. Another important effect is decrement of a neuropeptide, the brain-derived neurotropic factor (BDNF) in the brain, which is important for neuronal growth. Reduction in its concentration is responsible for loss of neurons in various regions of the brain.

Stress can also change cognition or the way we perceive the environment, analyse it and respond. Prefrontal cortex is the seat of cognition, whose activity is, in part, regulated by amygdala, which is the seat for emotions. A huge amount of literature has suggested that amygdala has a control over the prefrontal cortex and thus emotions can regulate the cognition. Thus, stress can change the way we perceive the environmental cues and in such situations they are usually given a negative valence, leading to distress. This negative valence further increases the perception of stress and a vicious cycle starts.

Whether the stress acts as a predisposing, precipitating or perpetuating factor for the psychiatric illness is not yet clearly known (please refer to unresolved issues). If stress were the *causative factor* for psychiatric illness, then all the persons who experience similar stress (amount, duration and also quality of stress) would have developed psychiatric illness, eg, all the soldiers who fought a war would have developed posttraumatic stress disorder (PTSD); all the people who suffered from a major catastrophe would have developed depression; all the persons who were stranded in a lift would have developed claustrophobia; and so on! But this does not happen. Thus, stress is not a *causative* or *aetiological* factor for any of the psychiatric disorders, at the most it may act as a *trigger* in persons having genetic predisposition for any of these illnesses. Does this mean that people who are genetically susceptible cannot tolerate stress at all or, in other words, they have low resilience? In these persons, can a trivial stress *trigger* psychiatric illness? This is difficult to answer at present owing to the lack of adequate data in this regard. Moreover, it is difficult to be tested in real world as resilience to stress is governed by multiple genetic factors (genes of various neurotransmitter receptors, eg, serotonin receptors; genes encoding enzymes that act on neurotransmitters, eg, allelic variation of catechol-*O*-methyl-transferase [COMT], to name a few) and also by learned behaviour owing to neuroplasticity of the brain.

RESILIENCE AND ADAPTATION TO STRESS

Whereas resilience to stress is in part genetic, still it may also be learned. It is shown in Fig. 3.6.1 that stress pathway is a closed loop. First step of the cascade is prefrontal cortex, which initiates the stress reaction and unfortunately bears a major brunt of stress. However, if we train our prefrontal cortex to deal with the stress, this reaction can be minimized or stopped at all which can be done through a variety of methods (Please refer to Chapter 9.1 on nonpharmacological therapies). Adaptation can also occur by the process of *extinction* when the inoculating doses of the stressors are given to a person.

IS STRESS ALWAYS BAD?

From what we have discussed so far, it appears that largely stress is bad for our health. But this notion is far from the truth. You are right now reading this book because you want to gather knowledge or you want to perform well in your examinations or in your clinical practice. We strive to achieve because we anticipate the stress arising out of failure that keeps our *engine* running and motivates us to work. Thus, some amount of stress is essential for growth. However, when it goes beyond the ability to adapt, it becomes distress and starts deteriorating our performance (Fig. 3.6.2).

UNRESOLVED ISSUES

1. All the symptoms that we see during acute or chronic stress (distress) are seen during stress-related disorders, in depression and in anxiety disorder. However, in these disorders, the symptoms are more severe, pervasive, last longer and, finally, they have some uncommon symptoms that help us to distinguish between them. On the other hand, in case of acute stress and distress, these symptoms reverse soon after the resolution of stressor in most patients. However, in some others, they may induce a widespread damage to neuronal networks and *manifest* the

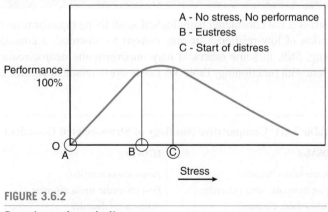

FIGURE 3.6.2

Stress is not always bad!

psychiatric disorder, a condition dependent upon the 'genetic' or 'biological' predisposition. However, how much part does stress play, whether it is major or minor, is still to be determined.

2. All the pathophysiological changes that we see during stress have been reported in various psychiatric disorders, eg, depression, PTSD, substance abuse, anxiety disorders and psychosis. There could be many reasons for it: first, their presence suggests shared neurobiological mechanisms between stress and psychiatric disorders; or there is a possibility that psychiatric illnesses themselves may be perceived as stressful by the brain, leading to recruitment of stress pathways. The latter hypothesis appears more appealing as successful treatment of psychiatric disorders have been found to reverse these changes.

3. It is also possible that the psychiatric illness-mediated stress changes the cognition, so that a person starts giving negative valence to usual life events. All of us experience a variety of negative life events everyday; hence, any of them can be picked by the patient and mistakenly considered as the aetiological factor for the development of psychiatric illness, eg, a patient may say that he/she developed depression after a major financial loss. Asking the patient whether he/she had experienced similar events during asymptomatic period as well, can test this! While doing so, please remember that owing to ongoing stress the patient may still attach a negative valence to life events.

4. Since we know that emotions also influence cognition, it is possible that during incipient stage of psychiatric illness, the individuals' cognition is changed in such a manner that they perceive the environment negatively. They then report stressor as the 'cause' of psychiatric illness.

TRAUMA AND STRESS-RELATED DISORDERS

Stress-related disorders are those conditions that appear immediately after a stress. These patients present with sympathetic arousal and behavioural changes (as explained in Fig. 3.6.1) along with the recall of stress or related memories.

NOSOLOGY

Normal day-to-day stress is not considered pathological as all living organisms on the earth experience it. However, in situation of low resilience, it may convert to 'distress', a condition that moderately affects the functioning. Still, in some others, it may uncover/ignite neurocircuitry to produce some symptoms that interfere with functioning. Table 3.6.1 lists stress-related disorders according to DSM-5 and ICD-10.

Table 3.6.1 Comparative Nosology of Stress-related Disorders

DSM-5	ICD-10
Acute stress disorder	Acute stress reaction
Post traumatic stress disorder	Post traumatic stress disorder
Adjustment disorder	Adjustment disorder

VIGNETTE

Mr. A, a 40-year-old man, presented with complaints of poor-quality sleep for 6 months. He reported that he wakes up at night after having bad dreams. He described that he met with a terrible accident 6 months back when he was going to some other place with his three friends in a car. On the highway, they met with an accident where two of his friends died on the spot and the third suffered major injuries. He was fortunate to have minimal injuries but had to manage everything till the rescue reached there. Since then he is not able to drive or sit in the car and now uses other means of transport, preferably a scooter or a bicycle. Almost every night, he re-experiences the same event in his dreams. He has become so fearful of sleep that even bedtime provokes anxiety. He often accuses himself for the death of his two friends. His wife noticed that he is not able to enjoy his work and becomes secluded and irritable since the accident. He and his wife noticed that symptoms started within 2–3 days of the event and continuing since then. On examination, vital signs were within normal limits. Examination of mental status showed pacing, apprehension on mention of the event; anxious mood and recurrent egodystonic thoughts of the trauma. Based on the history and examination, diagnosis of post traumatic stress disorder (PTSD) was made.

CLINICAL PICTURE

These disorders have symptoms from five major categories: (1) experiencing the trauma; (2) having recurrent intrusive memories or dreams of the event after having witnessed it; (3) avoidance to any kind of stimuli that can remind him of that event; (4) negative emotions associated with the event and, lastly, (5) a behavioural change after the event.

These patients often provide the history of having experienced a traumatic event (including sexual abuse) that endangered their life and/or inflicted serious injuries upon them. The event may be experienced in a variety of manners, eg, self-experiencing a car crash; or having eyewitnessed an event, eg, seeing a car banged into another; or that a close friend or relative has suffered a violent or accidental injury or has died during a violent accident; and, lastly, they may provide a history of repeated exposures to such events, eg, volunteers or persons who are engaged in relief work immediately after a disaster.

These people complain of recurrent memories of the episode that intrude with their consciousness. Some may report recurrent dreams of the incidence, whereas others may report having flashbacks, ie, re-experience the same event. An exposure to the cues that remind them of the event causes distress, eg, feeling distressed when look at an aircraft after witnessing 9/11.

These patients avoid, or at least attempt to avoid, persons, thoughts, places, tasks or any other kind of stimuli that may remind them of the event. For example, one may try to avoid sitting in any car; or try to avoid a car of similar make or design or colour which he/she had witnessed during accident.

In addition, these persons often develop a negative feeling towards themselves or others and may feel that either they are bad or that nobody in this world is reliable. These feelings often jeopardize their functioning. Some people may develop amnesia (please refer to Chapter 3.11 on dissociative disorders) and they are not able to recall even the important details of the event.

Behaviourally, these patients often remain in a state of hyperarousal and, consequently, they have all the behavioural manifestations of chronic stress, eg, poor concentration, irritability, sleep disturbance and amplified startle reflex.

Table 3.6.2 Trauma and Stress-Related Disorders in Adults

Category	Adjustment Disorder	Acute Stress Disorder	PTSD
Stressor	Never life threatening	Life threatening, serious injuries or sexual abuse	Life threatening, serious injuries or sexual abuse
Onset	Within 3 months of stressor	Within 3 days of stressor	Usually appear within 3 months of stressor but there may be a variable delay
Duration of symptoms	After termination of stressor, symptoms persists for a maximum of 6 months	Converts into PTSD after 1 month	Symptoms must be present for at least 1 month
Intrusive symptoms	May be present	Must be present	Must be present
Avoidance to stressor	Usually not seen	Must be present	Must be present
Hyperarousal	Not seen	Must be present	Must be present
Negative emotions and cognition	May be present	Must be present	Must be present
Course	Variable, depending upon the type and persistence of stressor; however, these patients are prone to suicide attempt and completed suicide	Variable	50% improvement within 3 months

If the symptoms start soon after the incidence and last for at least 3 days to a maximum of 30 days, it is termed as *acute stress reaction*. However, if the symptoms last longer than 1 month, it is known as PTSD (Table 3.6.2).

NEUROBIOLOGY

Patients with PTSD have abnormal response in the HPA axis. *Inherently*, they have increased negative feedback sensitivity of adrenocorticotrophic hormone (ACTH) to cortisol in addition to the reduction in numbers of corticotrophin releasing hormone (CRH) receptors in anterior pituitary (Fig. 3.6.3). This is why they have hypocortisolimia along with high concentration of CRH in cerebrospinal fluid at the time of exposure. Normally, cortisol inhibits the recall of fear-laden memories; however, in these patients hypocortisolimia disinhibits this system. To add to it, increased noradrenaline from the locus ceruleus and increased CRH in the brain increase the encoding of emotional and fear-laden memories, enhance the vigilance and augment the startle response (Figs. 3.6.1 and 3.6.3). Thus, PTSD patients have neurobiological vulnerability through a system that favours the encoding of fear-laden memories and disinhibited recall of traumatic events.

In these patients, the cortisol receptors on the hippocampus are thought to be hypersensitive, which even in the presence of hypocortisolimia, ensure degeneration of hippocampal neurons. Thus, anatomically, hippocampus gets atrophied. In functional terms, hypersensitivity of the hippocampal neurons to the cortisol increases the recall of fearful memories and leads to impaired negative feedback control of

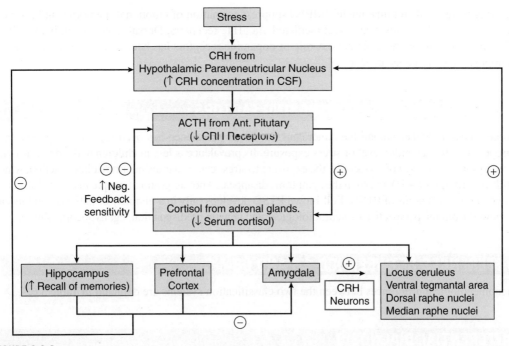

FIGURE 3.6.3

Neurobiology of PTSD.

paraventricular nuclei (Fig. 3.6.3). *This is a preexisting condition that makes one vulnerable to develop PTSD.*

Amygdala, though, does not show any structural abnormality in these patients, but it remains hyper-responsive and can be activated even by the trivial cues associated with the traumatic memories. That is why patients with PTSD develop symptoms when they are exposed to any cue that reminds him of the trauma.

PTSD is associated with the loss of neurons in prefrontal cortex and a reduction in their activity; however, it develops only after the appearance of symptoms. *Thus, neuronal loss in the prefrontal cortex in these patients is the effect of underlying pathology.* As we have already discussed earlier, reduced prefrontal activity disinhibits the amygdala, which initiates a cascade of events that produce symptoms akin to PTSD (Fig. 3.6.3).

Neurobiology of stress reaction will remain incomplete unless we discuss the role of monoamine nuclei. Amygdala projects to various monoaminergic nuclei via neurons that use CRH neuropeptide as the neurotransmitter. Due to hypocortisolimia and high CRH in the brain, these neurons remain in a state of hyperactivity. Due to overactivity of noradrenergic locus ceruleus, sympathetic system remains overactivated in these patients; thus, they are always prepared for the fight or flight response. Serotonergic raphe nuclei from the brainstem are also important in stress reactions. Dorsal raphe nuclei (DRN) projects to amygdala and to hippocampus and have anxiogenic effects via $5HT_2$ receptors. On the other hand, median raphe nuclei (MRN) suppress formation of emotional memories and promote their extinction (delearning), an effect mediated via $5HT_1$ receptors. Dorsal raphe nuceli is thought to have higher activity in these patients. A role of dopamine receptors has been found; however, its exact pathophysiology remains unclear.

EPIDEMIOLOGY AND PREDISPOSING FACTORS

Its prevalence is higher among the Americans but lower prevalence has been reported from Asia and Europe even after a similar level of stress exposure. Its prevalence is less in children and elderly as compared to adults. For most of the people, the exposure to stress causes a transient immediate reaction, which fulfils the criteria for ASD and soon the symptoms disappear. Another group of people may develop some, but not all the symptoms of PTSD. Full-blown PTSD develops only in a minority of patients and this can be viewed from the perspective of neurobiological and genetic predisposition, eg, hypocortisolimia.

DIFFERENCES BETWEEN ICD-10 AND DSM-5

Phenomenological differences between the two classification systems are depicted in Table 3.6.3.

DIFFERENTIAL DIAGNOSIS

It must be differentiated from adjustment disorder where trauma is less severe and type of stress can be different, eg, failure in examination or break-up. It is usually not life threatening. In adjustment disorder, the patients do not have symptoms from all five spheres, as explained above.

If the patients have episodes of sympathetic overactivity in the absence of other symptoms of PTSD, panic disorder should be diagnosed. Those who report avoidance to the stressor, phobia may be considered. Sometimes only amnesia for the event is seen and, in such cases, diagnosis of dissociative amnesia should be preferred.

Table 3.6.3 Differences in the ICD-10 Diagnosis from DSM-5

Adjustment Disorder	Acute Stress Reaction	PTSD
Symptoms start within 1 month of the stressor rather than 3 months, as specified in DSM-5.	Symptoms start within 1 h of exposure and begin to diminish within 48 h. Symptoms are similar to that of generalized anxiety disorder along with emotional symptoms as described in DSM-5. Intrusion, hyperarousal and avoidance are not required as in DSM-5.	Similar symptoms as in DSM-5 but should be seen within 6 months of exposure to stressor or termination of stressor. Duration of symptoms is not specified.

Thoughts in PTSD are intrusive and similar picture is also seen in patients with obsessive–compulsive disorder (OCD). However, a major stressor and other symptoms of PTSD are not seen in OCD.

In major depressive disorder, the mood is sad and other symptoms of PTSD are absent, as is the stressor.

DIAGNOSTIC FALLACIES

Diagnosis of these disorders rests on the objective severity and quality of stressor. However, emotional valence of any stressor varies from person to person and from time to time. Hence, sometimes what appears non-life threatening event to one, may be perceived as life threatening by the other. It may lead to missed or overdiagnosis of PTSD.

A wide difference in the prevalence of PTSD across continents raises the questions of clinical reliability of the diagnosis and raises the issue if it is related to the compensation. However, neurobiological studies confirm its entity as a clinical disorder. However, since the diagnosis is purely clinical, this must be differentiated from malingering.

Patients with traumatic brain injury may have similar symptoms. However, in these patients, cognitive decline is prominent along with less conspicuous emotional and behavioural symptoms. In these cases, diagnosis of PTSD should be considered only when the patient meets all the criteria of the disorder.

MANAGEMENT

Adjustment disorder usually responds to nonpharmacological therapies, eg, relaxation therapy and cognitive behaviour therapy (CBT). However, in cases with significant anxiety, benzodiazepines (eg, clonazepam 0.25–2 mg/day) for a short period may be prescribed; similarly, patients with depressive features may be started on antidepressants (eg, escitalopram 5–20 mg/day).

Management of ASD and PTSD can be divided into two categories: preventive and therapeutic. Both pharmacological and nonpharmacological therapies have been tried.

Recent evidences suggest that exogenous glucocorticoids soon after the stress can prevent or at least lessen the development of PTSD by the mechanisms mentioned above. Interestingly, benzodiazepines, which act on GABA receptors, do not have any preventive role in this disorder; rather they may worsen the symptoms. Thus, they should best be avoided. Among the nonpharmacological interventions, trauma-focused CBT and 'eye movement desensitization and reprocessing' (EMDR) have been found effective in the prevention of these disorders. As of now, we do not have literature to show the efficacy of counselling and debriefing as a preventive measure.

For the therapeutic purpose, CBT is advised for the treatment of PTSD among the nonpharmacological means. Prazosin (2–15 mg at bedtime), which interferes with noradrenergic neurotransmission, is effective for nightmares and improves the quality of sleep. Antidepressants acting on serotonin receptors are effective for mood and anxiety symptoms (sertraline 50–200 mg/day). Repetitive transcranial magnetic stimulation (r-TMS) has also been found effective in some studies.

COURSE AND PROGNOSIS

Kindly refer to Table 3.6.2 for course and prognosis.

SUMMARY

- Stress produces microstructural and functional changes in the brain that can initiate a cascade of events.
- Some amount of stress is essential for growth and facilitates learning.
- Stress can never cause, but, at the most, acts as a trigger to the psychiatric illness.
- ASD and PTSD develop only in a minority of persons who are exposed to extreme stress.
- CRH and HPA axis play pivotal role in development of these symptoms.
- Exogenous glucocorticoids can be helpful in preventing the development of PTSD.
- Selective serotonin reuptake inhibitors (SSRI) and alpha blockers are helpful in treatment of PTSD.

FURTHER READING

Stress

1. McEwen B. S. (2007). Physiology and Neurobiology of Stress and Adaptation: Central Role of the Brain. *Physiological Reviews*, 87:873–904.
2. McEwen B. S., Gray J. D., and Nasca C. (2015). Recognizing Resilience: Learning From the Effects of Stress on the Brain. *Neurobiology of Stress*, 1:1–11.
3. Okon-Singer H., Hendler T., Pessoa L., and Shackman A. J. (2015). The Neurobiology of Emotion-Cognition Interactions: Fundamental Questions and Strategies for Future Research. *Frontiers in Human Neuroscience* 9:58.
4. Southwick S. M., and Charney D. S. (2012). The Science of Resilience: Implications for the Prevention and Treatment of Depression. *Science*, 338:79–82.
5. Sudom K. A., Lee J. E., and Zamorski M. A. (2014). A Longitudinal Pilot Study of Resilience in Canadian Military Personnel. *Stress and Health*, 30:377–385.

Trauma and Stress Related Disorders

1. American Psychiatric Association. (2013). "Diagnostic and Statistical Manual of Mental Disorders." 5th edit, Author, Washington, DC.
2. Katzman M. A., Bleau P., Blier P., Chokka P., Kjernisted K., Van Ameringen M.; Canadian Anxiety Guidelines Initiative Group on behalf of the Anxiety Disorders Association of Canada/Association Canadienne does troubles anxieux and McGill University, Antony M. M., Bouchard S., Brunet A., Flament M., Grigoriadis S., Mendlowitz S., O'Connor K., Rabheru K., Richter P. M., Robichaud M., and Walker J.R. (2014). Canadian Clinical Practice Guidelines for the Management of Anxiety, Posttraumatic Stress and Obsessive-Compulsive Disorders. *BMC Psychiatry*, 14(Suppl 1):S1.
3. Koola M. M., Varghese S. P., and Fawcett J. A. (2014). High-Dose Prazosin for the Treatment of Post-traumatic Stress Disorder. *Therapeutic Advances in Psychopharmacology*, 4:43–47.
4. Sherin J. E., and Nemeroff C. B. (2011). Post-traumatic Stress Disorder: The Neurobiological Impact of Psychological Trauma. *Dialogues in Clinical Neuroscience*, 13(3):263–278.
5. Warner C. H., Warner C. M., Appenzeller G. N., and Hoge C. W. (2013). Identifying and Managing Posttraumatic Stress Disorder. *American Family Physician*, 88:827–834.
6. World Health Organization. (1992). "The ICD-10 Classification of Mental and Behavioural Disorders: Clinical Descriptions and Diagnostic Guidelines." Author, Geneva.
7. http://www.ptsd.va.gov/professional/treatment/overview/clinicians-guide-to-medications-for-ptsd.asp (accessed 1 Nov 2015).

SEXUAL DISORDERS

3.7

Sex is considered as one of the basic needs and is important for procreation so as to maintain the existence of a species. It is a complex physiological activity, which involves multiple areas of the brain, peripheral nervous system, sexual organs and, lastly, the hormones. Interaction between so many systems of the body predisposes this activity to go disordered in some persons. Thus, sexual disorders are those disorders that present with the recurrent interference in normal sexual act. These difficulties arise due to problem in one or more of the phases of normal sexual response cycle (SRS) that are regulated by coordinated activity of organ systems mentioned above. However, difficulties arising due to grossly conspicuous anatomical (damage to genitalia) or environmental problems (issues related to the relationship of the couple) are not included under this rubric.

NOSOLOGY

There is some difference in the nomenclature used in DSM-5 and ICD-10. This is depicted in Table 3.7.1.

Table 3.7.1 Comparative Nosology of Sexual Disorders	
DSM-5	**ICD-10**
Male hypoactive sexual desire disorder	Lack or loss of sexual desire
Female sexual interest/desire disorder	
Erectile disorder	Failure of genital response
Premature ejaculation	Premature ejaculation
Delayed ejaculation	–
Genitopelvic pain/penetration disorder	Nonorganic dysperunia
Female orgasmic disorder	Orgasmic dysfunction

VIGNETTE

A 27-year-old married man presented with history of early ejaculation for the past 6 months. He has been married for 8 months and is experiencing this difficulty since then. According to him, his wife is not satisfied (never achieved orgasm) and has started complaining about it since the past 6 months. Now he is afraid of indulging in sexual activity and remains preoccupied with the thought of sexual inadequacies. This is affecting his work performance and he makes mistakes frequently. Because of this, his emotional relationship with his wife has also deteriorated. He has reported that he achieves erection while he watches any movie with sensual scenes and appears to have desire for sexual activity. There is no history to suggest substance abuse, medical disorders or psychiatric disorders. General physical examination showed that vital signs were within normal limits. Mental status examination showed distressed mood and preoccupation with the inability to perform sexual act. Based on the history and examination, diagnosis of premature ejaculation was made.

CLINICAL PICTURE

The symptoms vary from disorder to disorder and all the disorders have different symptoms. In *male hypoactive sexual desire disorder*, the patient does not have any desire to indulge in sexual activity, which is accompanied by the absence of erotic fantasies and lack of sexual thoughts that persist for at least 6 months. This problem may be lifelong or may appear after a period of normal sexual activity. Furthermore, it can be limited to one type of situation or a specific partner or may be generalized.

On the contrary, *female sexual interest/desire disorder* does not limit to the thoughts and desires as we see in male hypoactive sexual desire disorder. Women, in addition to symptoms mentioned above, show either reduction or complete loss in initiation of sexual activity. There perception of sexual activity is also altered and they are not able to appreciate the genital and extragenital stimulation. Even if the activity is initiated, they are not able to feel the pleasure, another component of perception.

Erectile disorder is seen in males and is characterized by difficulty in either achieving an erection or maintaining it or by a reduction in the stiffness. These problems must be seen on at least 75% sexual attempts and symptoms must be present for at least 6 months. In some patients, this problem may be lifelong, whereas in others, it may appear after a period of normal sexual activity. Furthermore, it can be limited to one type of situation or to a specific partner. However, in other cases, it may be generalized.

Genitopelvic pain/penetration disorder is seen among females and is characterized by a marked pain in the vulvovaginal region during penetration that makes the penetration difficult. Woman may have anticipatory anxiety of this pain leading to avoidance of the act. Symptoms must persist for at least 6 months. This problem may be lifelong or may appear after a period of normal sexual activity.

Premature ejaculation is seen in males only and is defined as ejaculation within 1 min of vaginal penetration or before it is desired. Symptoms must be persistent for at least 6 months and must be experienced on at least 75% attempts. This problem may be lifelong or may appear after a period of normal sexual activity. Furthermore, it can be limited to one type of situation or to a specific partner or may be generalized. Similarly, *delayed ejaculation* is characterized by infrequent or absence of ejaculation or a delay in ejaculation that is seen on at least 75% sexual attempts and symptoms are present even when the male does not want them, for at least 6 months.

Female orgasmic disorder is characterized by either a delay or infrequent experiences of orgasms. In some patients, there may be a complete absence of an orgasm. Other patients may report a reduction in its intensity. These symptoms must be present on at least 75% of sexual acts and for at least 6 months. This problem may be lifelong or may appear after a period of normal sexual activity. Furthermore, it can be limited to one type of situation or with a specific partner; in some cases it may be generalized.

However, before making a diagnosis of any of these conditions, kindly ensure that symptoms are not the effect of any substance of abuse, not related to any medication, are not because of the relationship issues and cannot be better explained by any other psychiatric or medical disorders.

NEUROBIOLOGY

It is important for you to understand the normal neurobiology of the sexual act as these disorders emerge from a dysfunction in this system. In this chapter, we will focus only on the emotional part of sexual acts.

DIFFERENCE BETWEEN LOVE AND SEXUAL DESIRE

Feelings of love and the sexual desire as well, activate a large number of brain areas that include ventral tegmental area (dopamine pathway), amygdala (emotion), ventral striatum, hypothalamus (hormones, autonomic nervous system, vital activity), thalamus and a number of cortical areas, eg, insula (social cues), anterior cingulate gyrus (motivation), middle frontal gyrus, superior central and precentral gyrus (body language), temporoparietal area, somatosensory cortex (perception) and insula (visceral integration). These areas help in understanding the body language, emotions of other people and social cues. In addition, they convey the sensory stimuli and anticipate the feeling of reward. Thus, the feeling of love and sexual desire have overlapping network; however, both the acts differ with the fact that during the feeling of love, anterior parts of the insula gets activated, and during sexual desire, posterior part of the insula gets activated.

Functional neuroimaging has disclosed a low activity in amygdala, ventral striatum, hypothalamus, inferior parietal lobule and somatosensory cortex during the feeling of love, which suggests that it is an abstract feeling. Feeling of love is associated with a high-activity dorsal striatum, one region that is highly dopaminergic (receives dopaminergic neurons from ventral tegmental area as well as substantia nigra). This is involved in reward expectancy and habit formation. On the other hand, sexual desire evokes activity in ventral striatum that receives dopaminergic signals from ventral tegmental area only (Fig. 3.7.1). Thus, love and lust are, though overlapping, but still different, even neurobiologically. It also conveys the notion that emotions play an important role in sexual activity.

SEXUAL RESPONSE CYCLE

Human SRC starts consist of a variety of phases. First phase is the desire, ie, one must be motivated for the act of copulation. This desire depends upon a variety of issues—what do the social norms guide about being engaged with a partner; qualities of the stimuli that evoke desire (stimulus can be a partner whom one loves or can be the pornographic material; other important characters are novelty of stimuli, appearance of the partner and, ambience), one's emotional state (stressed mind cannot have sexual desire), past experiences with the sexual acts and, lastly, physical state of the person.

Having this desire in the brain, in the appropriate sexual context, one feels excited with the engorgement of genitalia. This constructs the second phase of SRS and is known as consummation phase.

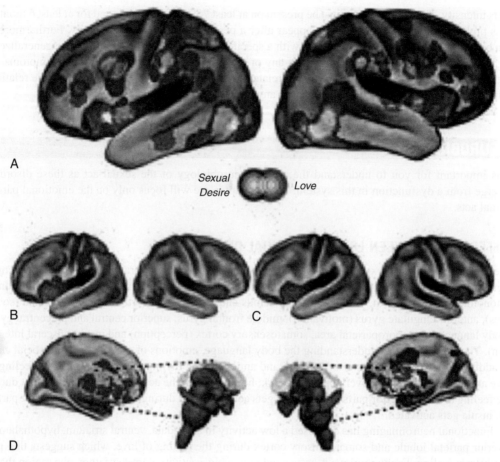

FIGURE 3.7.1

Areas involved in sexual desire versus love. (A) Note that many areas are overlapping. (B) Dorsolateral cortical areas activated during sexual desires. (C) Dorsolateral cortical areas activated during feeling of love. (D) Medial side of the brain and brainstem.

(Source: *Cacioppo S, Bianchi-Demicheli F, Frum C, Pfaus JG, Lewis JW. The common neural bases between sexual desire and love: A multilevel kernel density fMRI analysis. J Sex Med 2012;9:1048–1054.)*

After being engaged in the sexual act for some time, while excitation remains on a plateau, one reaches orgasm with ejaculation. With orgasm, one enters the third phase of SRS—the satiety phase. After an orgasm, males usually have a refractory period (Fig. 3.7.2).

Now we will discuss all the phases of SRC phase one by one in detail.

First phase—desire

Desire is initiated by a number of stimuli from our special senses. We have five special senses—smell, taste, hearing, touch and vision. It *appears* that in humans the olfaction can potentiate the sexual desire,

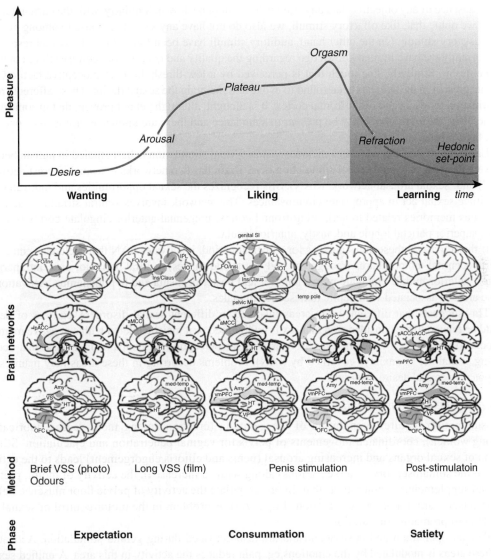

FIGURE 3.7.2

Brain activity during various phases of the SRS. Light-blue colour indicates high activity, whereas dark blue shows reduction in activity.

(Source: Georgiadis JR, Kringelbach ML. The human sexual response cycle: Brain imaging evidence linking sex to other pleasures. Progress in Neurobiology 2012;98:49–81.)

but in absence of any objective data any conclusion cannot be drawn. Similarly, with the current knowledge, we opine that, like olfactory stimuli, we also do not have any sexual response to among humans the gustatory stimuli. On the other hand, auditory stimuli have been found to evoke sexual responses, but currently we have limited knowledge regarding the quality and quantity of auditory stimuli that can evoke desire. Similarly, fine touch that is perceived by a low-threshold mechanoceptive tactile C afferents present in the skin has been found to evoke and maintain the sexual desire. These afferents relay information to insula and orbitofrontal cortex. It is thought, although yet not proven, that in some areas of the body, these receptors may be present in abundance and these are known as erotogenic zones,eg, lips, face, nipples and genitalia.

Last category of special senses includes vision. Visual stimulation is best studied in human beings, so we will focus on visual sexual stimulation here. Brain has two networks—'sexual interest network' (SIN) and 'sexual arousal network' (SAN). SIN recognizes the sexual opportunities and motivates one to initiate sexual act in appropriate circumstances. This network involves ventral striatum, amygdala (previous memories related to act), orbitofrontal cortex, pregenual anterior cingulate cortex (motivation), superior parietal lobule and, lastly, anterior insula.

If the activity in these areas persists for a critical period, it activates SAN that includes ventral and lateral occipital-temporal area (recognizes body parts and shapes), ventral premotor area, intraparietal cortex, anterior middle cingulate gyrus, anterior and posterior insula and hypothalamus. Activation of these areas is associated with penile tumescence in males.

This suggests that different brain areas involved in different sexual disorders, eg, loss of desire could be related to the consideration that sex is undignified or it may be related with a negative memory associated with the act (governed by SIN) or with misperception of sympathetic arousal that occurs during sexual act as anxiety (governed by SAN). Problems occurring in these areas may manifest as 'hypoactive sexual desire disorders'.

Second phase—consummation

Consummation requires preparation of the genitalia (erection among men; vaginal lubrication among women), coordinated movements of pelvis for vaginal penetration and ejaculation. Stimulation of sexual organs and increasing arousal (penis and clitoris engorgement) leads to the activation of the somatosensory area (sensations) along with an increase in the activity of motor, premotor and supplementary motor areas that, in turn, regulate the activity of pelvic floor muscles. Pelvic floor muscles are important for erection (Fig. 3.7.3). A problem in the motor control of sexual act can lead to premature ejaculation.

Parietal operculum and posterior insula are also activated during genital stimulation. Activation of these areas is modulated by the emotions,eg, pain reduces the activity in this area. A unified sexual experience requires information from three different areas. First, emotional information from the medial temporal cortex; second, information from the frontal motor area and third, information from the parietal operculum. Thus, sexual act requires coordination between emotions and motor activity.

Penile erection is associated with high activity in posterior insula and claustrum. However, in women this area is less-acting and this suggests that men are more aware of penile erection than women regarding their clitoral engorgement. This also shows why erectile dysfunction is an important aspect of male sexual dysfunction.

Once the sexual activity is started, it is maintained by high activity in the SAN. Even when the partner stops stimulating the genitalia, this activity continues through a self-referential processing

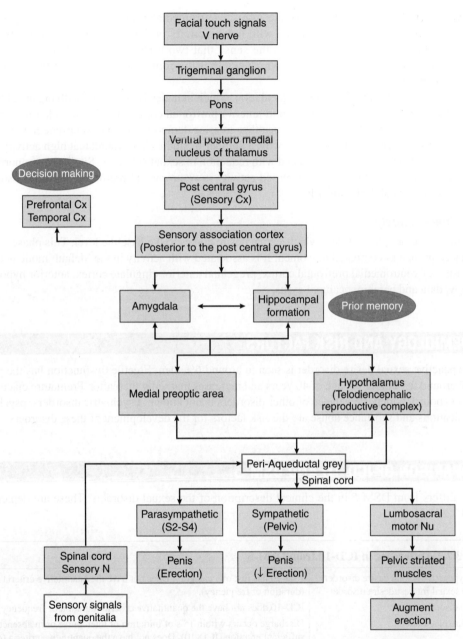

FIGURE 3.7.3

Neuroanatomy of sexual activity.

that involves pregenual anterior cingulate gyrus, ventromedial prefrontal cortex, amygdala and parahippocampal area. This is associated with lower activity in the amygdala. Low activity in the amygdala reduces alertness and provides the sense that two bodies are indeed one. At the same time, vermis of the cerebellum activates which signifies the coordinated activity of the pelvic contractions during the sexual act.

Continuation of this activity leads to ejaculation, which in males is associated with orgasm. Orgasm is associated with lowered activity in the mid-anterior prefrontal cortex that signifies pleasure and loss of inhibition. Besides this specific area, some other areas,eg, temporal lobe and ventromedial prefrontal cortex, also show reduced activity. This is why, a number of studies have found that high activity in the mid-anterior prefrontal cortex is associated with reduction in sexual activities. Similarly, temporal lobe damage leads to hypersexuality and increased activity in ventromedial prefrontal cortex is associated with hypoactive sexual desire disorder.

Phase three—satiety

This is the refractory phase during which sexual desire comes to the baseline level. This phase is more pronounced in men as compared to women. It is associated with activity in the 'default mode network' that consists of ventromedial prefrontal cortex, pregenual anterior cingulate cortex, anterior hypothalamus, amygdala and parahippocampal gyrus.

EPIDEMIOLOGY AND RISK FACTORS

Male hypoactive sexual desire disorder is seen in around 6% men. Erectile dysfunction has the prevalence of around 2% before the age of 40 years and increases markedly thereafter. Premature ejaculation is seen in about 1% men. Prevalence of other disorders is not known. Psychiatric disorders, psychotropic medications and substance abuse are the risk factors for the development of these disorders.

COMPARISON OF ICD-10 AND DSM-5

ICD-10 differs from DSM-5 in the clinical description of the sexual disorders. These are depicted in Table 3.7.2.

Table 3.7.2 Difference in ICD-10 from DSM-5

Male hypoactive sexual desire disorder Female sexual interest/desire disorder	ICD-10 has just one category. Does not have the quantitative criteria (duration or frequency).
Erectile disorder	ICD-10 does not have the quantitative criteria (duration or frequency).
Premature ejaculation	Discharge occurs within 15 s of initiation of intercourse or in absence of sufficient erection (ICD-10). Does not have the quantitative criteria (duration or frequency).
Genitopelvic pain/penetration disorder	Viginusmus to be excluded (ICD-10). Does not have the quantitative criteria (duration or frequency).
Female orgasmic disorder	Does not have the quantitative criteria (duration or frequency).

DIFFERENTIAL DIAGNOSIS

These disorders must be differentiated from one another. Psychiatric and other medical disorders may present with these symptoms, so they should be ruled out before diagnosing these disorders.

These disorders must be differentiated from adverse effects of neuropsychotropic substances including medications.

DIAGNOSTIC FALLACIES

These disorders should best be diagnosed when the couple is present. Remember, sexual activity involves two partners and problem in one partner may emerge as the problem in other, eg, a lady with orgasmic disorder may report the same to her partner and the partner may mistakenly consider it as premature ejaculation. Similarly, consider another situation where poor cooperation from the lady who is suffering from hypoactive desire disorder may lead to erectile dysfunction in male.

Sometimes, a male complaining of erectile dysfunction may actually have hypoactive sexual desire disorder. Thus, a thoughtful history taking is important while diagnosing sexual disorders.

MANAGEMENT

Management of sexual disorder varies with the diagnosis. The management can be nonpharmacological or pharmacological. Nonpharmacological management includes relaxation technique; for premature ejaculation, the male may be taught 'squeeze technique' (tightly squeezing the penis during the act when it is rigid, so that it becomes flaccid and the act may be restarted).

Pharmacological management includes use of selective serotonin reuptake inhibitors for premature ejaculation (paroxetine 12.5 mg before the act). Erectile dysfunction may be addressed using sildenafil (25–50 mg before the act).

COURSE AND PROGNOSIS

Most of these disorders are amenable to treatment. However, little is known about their course.

SUMMARY

- Sexual disorders are common; however, their presentation depends upon gender.
- These disorders arise owing to a variety of factors; hence, comprehensive history taking is important.
- One sexual disorder may pave the way for another.
- They are amenable to appropriate treatment.

FURTHER READING

1. American Psychiatric Association. (2013). "Diagnostic and Statistical Manual of Mental Disorders." 5th edit, Author, Washington, DC.
2. Cacioppo S., Bianchi-Demicheli F., Frum C., Pfaus J. G., and Lewis J. W. (2012). The Common Neural Bases Between Sexual Desire and Love: A Multilevel Kernel Density fMRI Analysis. *The Journal of Sex Medicine*, 9:1048–1054.
3. Georgiadis J. R., and Kringelbach M. L. (2012). The Human Sexual Response Cycle: Brain Imaging Evidence Linking Sex to Other Pleasures. *Progress in Neurobiology*, 98:49–81.
4. Kim S. W.,Schenck C. H., Grant J. E., Yoon G., Dosa P. I., Odlaug B. L., Schreiber L. R. N., Hurwitz T. D., and Pfaus J. G. (2013). Neurobiology of Sexual Desire. *NeuroQuantology*, 11:332–359.
5. World Health Organization. (1992). "The ICD-10 Classification of Mental and Behavioural Disorders: Clinical Descriptions and Diagnostic Guidelines." Author, Geneva.

PERSONALITY DISORDERS

3.8

Ravi Gupta

Personality can be defined as a set of behaviour and emotions that are enduring, pervasive and woven into a person to that extent that the whole of the functioning of the given person is regulated by them. This is also considered as the 'characteristic' of the person by which he/she is recognized, eg, friendly, ignorant, strict, 'by the books', introvert and so on! These behaviours (acts) and emotions (ie, how they feel) do not change over time (ie, enduring) and often guide the person's behaviour into any given context (ie, pervasive). For example, an introvert person, even while going through a situation that is sufficient to provoke euphoria in others, despite feeling pleasure to same extent, does not become as 'outgoing' as an extrovert person. Opposite would happen to an extrovert person during the time of low mood. In psychiatry practice, where we are dealing with behavioural alterations, knowledge of personality is extremely important because it can modify the clinical manifestations of the psychiatric disorders, as exemplified above. However, unless these characteristics are deviant, until they induce distress into a person's life, by that time they are not considered disorders. Thus, personality disorders are those enduring and pervasive patterns of behaviour and emotions that are deviant from the social and cultural norms to the extent that the person develops distress because of them and, despite the distress, remain inflexible.

NOSOLOGY

There are differences between the nomenclature of personality disorders between DSM-5 and ICD-10. These are outlined in Table 3.8.1.

VIGNETTE

Ms X, 28-year-old woman, was brought to the psychiatry OPD because she was not able to continue her job at any place. She had completed her masters in management studies and appeared to be a good student; yet her colleagues at any of her workplaces place did not seem to like her.

In 2 years she changed five jobs, all in multinational companies and from each place she had to resign because of social and emotional problems. Being involved in such frequent job changes, now no company is ready to hire her. When she was brought, she appeared distressed and she cried many times during the course of examination. Her mother communicated that she had unstable relationships since her adolescence with her friends, both boys and girls. Ms X conveyed that 'everybody used her' and she did not have any 'real friend' in her life. Whenever she realized that her friends were using her, she confronted them and often became verbally and physically abusive to them. After such incidences they left her and on every such occasion she slashed her wrists to save her relationship. She confirmed that she had never experienced true love in her life and her heart has always remained empty. She communicated that even her parents do not love her the way they should. Her mother communicated that her relationships were short-lasting because she used to be 'sticky' to her friends, even after a short period of friendship and started 'expecting a lot'. When the other people were not able to provide that much attention, she felt dejected and often started blaming them. General physical examination was within normal limits except for the hesitation marks (Fig. 3.8.1). Mental status examination showed anxiety, distress and guilt. Based on the clinical history and examination, diagnosis of borderline personality disorder was made.

CLINICAL PICTURE

Clinical picture varies with each case. Please refer to Tables 3.8.2–3.8.4 to understand the clinical picture of each of these disorders. In general, these behavioural patterns arc conspicuous by adolescence and they colour all aspects of the person's life. These patients do not have any overt symptom as seen in some other psychiatric disorders. Rather, they present with subtle problems that cause distress in day-to-day functioning. All of us have these traits but we do not label the disorder unless they are the source of distress or dysfunction. Personality disorders can grossly be divided into three categories–clusters A, B and C. Cluster A has 'odd-eccentric' personality; cluster B are 'emotional and dramatic' and those belonging to cluster C are 'anxious and fearful'.

Table 3.8.1 Comparative Nosology of Personality Disorders

DSM-5	ICD-10
Paranoid personality disorder	Paranoid personality disorder
Schizoid personality disorder	–
Schizotypal personality disorder	(included in schizophrenia and other psychotic disorders)
Antisocial personality disorder	Dissocial personality disorder
Borderline personality disorder	Emotionally unstable personality disorder
	Impulsive type
	Borderline type
Histrionic personality disorder	Histrionic personality disorder
Narcissistic personality disorder	–
Avoidant personality disorder	Anxious (avoidant) personality disorder
Dependent personality disorder	Dependent personality disorder
Obsessive compulsive personality disorder	Anankastic personality disorder

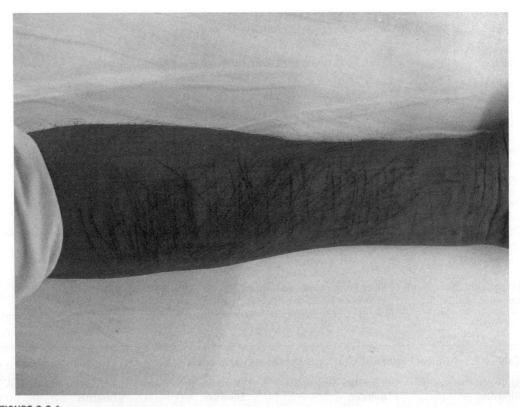

FIGURE 3.8.1

Hesitation marks in the forearm.

(Source: *Himalayan Hospital, Dehradun*)

People with cluster A show unusual behaviours; they possess feelings and emotions that do not go along with social beliefs; they do not enjoy relationships; harbour odd thinking, eg, paranoia without any reason; or magical beliefs, eg, they can control others. They are not able to express their emotions that connect them with the people or show extremely negative emotions. Emotionally, they may be indifferent to others, or feel that others are trying to make fun of them. This category includes paranoid personality disorder, schizoid personality disorder and schizotypal personality disorder.

Persons with cluster B are extremely emotional but have frequently changing emotions that make them unpredictable. They may be callous to the feelings of others and have extreme sense of superiority. They always want to be the centre of attraction. They are impulsive and take decisions that do not stand the test of time. They may be deceitful for personal gains. They throw their charm on others to initiate the relationship but are not able to maintain them. It includes antisocial personality disorder, borderline personality disorder, histrionic personality disorder and narcissistic personality disorder.

Persons with cluster C characters always feel anxious, they are dependent on other, need constant 'push' and appreciation to continue their work, keep on searching for new 'anchor points' and go by the rule book. This category has avoidant personality disorder, dependent personality disorder and obsessive–compulsive personality disorder.

Table 3.8.2 Clinical Picture of Cluster A Personality Disorders

Paranoid Personality Disorder	Schizoid Personality Disorder	Schizotypal Personality Disorder
Suspicious often without any evidence Always doubt loyalty of friends without any evidence Have difficulty in relying on others Try to find hidden messages in general remarks Bear grudges for long time React quickly and angrily Often doubts the fidelity of spouse	Do not enjoy close relationships, even in family Prefer solitary activities Do not enjoy sexual pleasures Do not find any activity pleasurable Do not have close friends Criticism and praise by others do not affect them Emotionally cold and do not show affect	Ideas of reference but never delusions Magical thinking—believes in superstition, sixth sense Odd perceptual experiences related to daily acts, eg., somebody else is doing an act because they commanded others to do it through telepathy Odd thinking and speech, eg, talk contains phrases that are idiosynchratic Paranoid ideas Inappropriate affect and not able to show all emotions Eccentric behaviour, not able to easily mingle with others, wear clothes that are 'out of context' Social anxiety: not able to communicate well; thus, have few friends, if any
In the United States, prevalence is around 2–4%	In the United States, prevalence in between 3–5%	In the United States, prevalence is between 0.6% and 5%.

Table 3.8.3 Clinical Picture of Cluster B Personality Disorders

Antisocial Personality Disorder	Borderline Personality Disorder	Histrionic Personality Disorder	Narcissistic Personality Disorder
Persistently defy the law Persistently deceitful Takes impulsive decisions Repeatedly engaged in fights and assaults Do not care for safety of themselves or others Irresponsible behaviours both at work place and in financial transactions e.g., not keeping up the time or impulsive expenditure Do not repent even after hurting others Conduct disorder must be present before the age of 15 years Age at diagnosis should be at least 18 years	Not able to tolerate perceived or real relinquishment Unstable personal relationships Markedly disturbed self-image Impulsive acts related to sexual activity, substance abuse, eating in binges or spending money Recurrent suicidal acts Marked changes in emotions that do not last more than a few days Always feel 'empty' inside Difficulty controlling anger Develop paranoid ideations or dissociative symptoms during periods of stress	Always try to be the centre of attraction Show emotions that shift rapidly Use their appearance to draw attention Dramatize Often use impressive words during communication but are not able to provide reason for the same Can be easily influenced by situations or by others Overvalue the intimacy of relationship than they actually are	Always feel themselves more important than others Always fantasizes about success, achievements and talents Believe that they are unique and special Always require admiration Always feel that they deserve special treatment Exploit others for their benefits Lack empathy Always envy other or feel that others are jealous Arrogant in behaviour
In the United States, prevalence is between 0.2% and 3.3%	In the United States, prevalence is between 1.6% and 6%; among psychiatric in-patients, it can be as high as 20%	In the United States, prevalence is 1.9%	In the United States, prevalence is between 0 and 6.2%

Table 3.8.4 Clinical Picture of Cluster C Personality Disorders

Avoidant Personality Disorder	Dependent Personality Disorder	Obsessive–compulsive Personality Disorder
Always fearful of criticism; hence, avoid team activities Make sure that others like them, otherwise avoid involving with others Always feel that they will be rejected by others Not able to start new relations because they feel the inadequacy Consider themselves inferior to others Reluctant to take personal risks	Always require reassurances to make decisions Want others to take responsibility for major areas of their life Have difficulty in showing disagreement Lack confidence to start any project Can submit themselves to any extent to get nurturance Extremely uncomfortable when they are alone Always need a relationship Unrealistic fears that they are not able to take care of themselves	Unrealistically follow the rules and regulations Not able to complete the tasks because they want it to be done perfectly Work on the cost of leisure activities even when not required Inflexible with regards to morality and ethics Not able to discard objects Not able to delegate tasks unless they do it the way they like it Miserly spending Rigid and stubborn behaviour
In the United States, prevalence is 2.4%	In the United States, prevalence varies between 0.5% and 0.6%	In the United States, prevalence varies between 2% and 8%

NEUROBIOLOGY

Neurobiology of personality is not as straightforward as we think it is, because of the number of factors that act together to give it a shape. Simplistically speaking, you are born with a brain carrying certain genes that regulate the release of neurotransmitters in your brain. This action of neurotransmitters across different brain areas regulates our perception, feeling and emotions. However, brain is plastic and we keep on learning new skills and concepts throughout our life. This learning changes the neurotransmission in the brain and thus, modifies our emotions and behaviour. Thus, both nature and nurture play a role in the development of our personality. If we deconstruct the personality, it can be divided into three entities—temperaments, character and psyche (Fig. 3.8.2).

TEMPERAMENT

Temperament regulates 'how' we react to the environment in different situations and manifests early in life. Thus, it is inheritable. Four different traits consist our temperament and we possess all of them, but in varying proportions. These temperamental traits are harm avoidance, novelty seeking, reward dependence and persistence.

People with high *harm avoidance* are fearful and anxious, whereas those with low harm avoidance are daring and optimistic. Exploration and impulsivity are seen in those with high *novelty seeking*, whereas those who are 'low' of this trait are reserved and apathetic. High *reward dependence* makes you sentimental and affectionate,whereas its low proportion makes you cold and independent. Lastly, people with high *persistence* are perfectionist and industrious, whereas those having low of it are

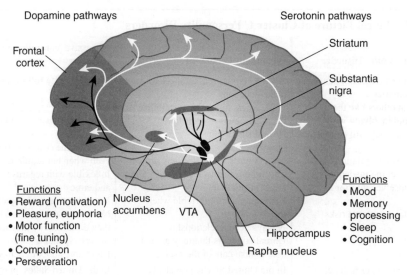

FIGURE 3.8.2

Neurobiological mechanisms of personality disorders.

(Source: https://appsychtextbk.wikispaces.com/file/view/Dopamine_and_serotonin_pathways_(1).gif/272112952/504x336/Dopamine_and_serotonin_pathways_(1).gif)

lazy and underachiever. Though these traits help you to adapt to the environment, but sometimes they become maladaptive (Table 3.8.5).

Thus, a person who has high novelty seeking, high harm avoidance and low reward dependence is at a high risk for the development of borderline personality disorder, whereas one with high novelty seeking, low harm avoidance and low reward dependence is at a high risk for antisocial personality disorder. Temperamental traits influence learning, and thus we develop different characters.

CHARACTER

Character is the one that we learn from the environment and it regulates secondary emotions, eg, empathy, patience, faith and hope. Since it is learned, it develops after we start understanding the external world. Understanding the environment, in turn, requires abstraction, reasoning and symbolic interpretation. Thus, to develop the character we require matured neocortex and hippocampus. The information lying in these areas interacts with the temperament traits and this interaction provides us the concept regarding self and about others. Thus, we learn to govern ourselves, and three discrete character traits emerge—self-directedness, cooperativeness and self-transcendence. A person with high self-directedness is responsible, reliable, self-sufficient and goal oriented. On the other hand, those with low self-directedness are blaming, reactive, unreliable and not responsible. Cooperativeness makes us a part of the society; persons with high cooperativeness are empathetic and supportive, whereas those with low cooperativeness are critical, unhelpful and opportunistic. Self-transcendence governs the quality of making us a part of the universe. People with high self-transcendence consider

Table 3.8.5 Temperamental Traits: Functions and Neurobiology

Trait	Proportion	Behavioural Effect		Neurotransmitter	Anatomy
		Adaptive	Maladaptive		
Harm avoidance	High	Promotes careful planning during anticipated danger	Induces apprehension and behavioural reticence even when danger is anticipated but unlikely to occur	Gamma amino butyric acid (GABA) and serotonin	Dorsal raphe nuclei and GABA neurons
	Low	Makes you cheerful, relaxed and confident even in those situations, which make most of the people nervous	Makes you unrealistically sanguine and do not prepare for the danger		
Novelty seeking	High	Promotes exploration in new environment. They are innovative and original	People easily gets uninterested in any task, are irritable and impulsive	Dopamine	Mesolimbic and mesocortical dopaminergic tracts
	Low	Makes you easily tolerate monotony and impassive	Makes you less enthusiastic and exploratory		
Reward dependence	High	Promotes sociability, sympathetic, dependable	Causes loss of self and encourages suggestibility	Norepinephrine Serotonin	Locus ceruleus Dorsal raphe nuclei
	Low	Makes you independent and enhances 'selfness'so that you arenot easily influenced by others	Induces social withdrawal, unimotional and aloof from the society		
Persistence	High	Promotes tireless working, do not require any reinforcement to keep working, focused on the work even during situations inducing frustration	It becomes maladaptive when the work requires frequent shifting of means to do the work	Glutamate Serotonin	Dorsal raphe nuclei
	Low	Makes you unstable, intolerant to the adverse environment and promotes sluggishness and torpor	Makes you less adaptive to situations where you need to work hard for a long time to get reward		

themselves a part of the universe, are humble, insightful and spiritual. People with low self-transcendence are materialistic and controlling. *The character regulates the expression of the temperamental traits.* In other words, epigenetic phenomenon can alter the expression of message incorporated in genes. Thus, a person with high novelty seeking and low harm avoidance will become antisocial or borderline personality if he has low self-directedness and low cooperativeness or a scientist if he has high self-directedness and high cooperativeness.

PSYCHE

It refers to the awareness of self in the world. It depends upon the episodic memory that rests in the prefrontal cortex. It has five levels, each more complex than the earlier one and, with maturity, one grows through these levels. At first, it promotes the feeling about the existence of oneself. Then, it makes you realize that there is freedom and that you can move ahead with time. On the next level, it provides you a sense of what is loveable and beautiful and has to be admired, both animate and inanimate objects. Fourth, it helps you to understand the absolute truth. Lastly, it makes you experience that everyone is good and needs to be admired.

To conclude, interplay of three factors, temperament, character and psyche, helps us to understand and to respond to the world. This complex interplay is also responsible for a unique shape to our personality.

Personality disorders result from the deviation in any of these systems. In summary, personality profile depends upon the genes that regulate temperament, anatomical and physiological maturation of brain areas so that we develop character and psyche. This explains why drugs are effective in personality disorders, why brain injury changes the personality and, lastly, why some of the psychiatric illness are associated with a particular personality type.

EPIDEMIOLOGY AND RISK FACTORS

Prevalence of various personality disorders is mentioned in Tables 3.8.2–3.8.4. As far as the risk factors are concerned, family members of schizophrenia patients are at high risk for paranoid personality disorder, schizoid personality disorder and schizotypal personality disorder.

Antisocial personality disorder is more common among family members of antisocial personality disorder. Similarly, borderline personality disorders increases the risk of having it in biological relatives.

DIFFERENCES BETWEEN ICD-10 AND DSM-5

ICD-10 differs from DSM-5 in certain aspects of personality disorders, as outlined in Table 3.8.6.

DIFFERENTIAL DIAGNOSIS

Paranoid personality disorder must be differentiated from other psychotic disorders. Schizoid personality disorder must be differentiated from autistic spectrum disorder. Schizotypal personality disorder must be differentiated from other psychotic disorders and neurodevelopmental disorders.

Table 3.8.6 Difference in ICD-10 from DSM-5

ICD-10 Mentions Following Additional Symptoms	
Paranoid personality disorder	Excessive self-importance
Schizoid personality disorder	Most of the activities do not provide pleasure
	Appear insensitive to prevailing social norms
Antisocial personality disorder	Not able to maintain relationships
	Always blame others
	Conduct disorder is not a prerequisite for the diagnosis
Borderline personality disorder	No difference
Histrionic Personality disorder	No difference
Obsessive–compulsive personality disorder	Overcautious
Avoidant personality disorder	Need physical security to the extent that they restrict their lifestyle
Dependent personality disorder	Not able to make reasonable demands to those, on whom they are dependent

Antisocial personality disorder should be differentiated from substance use because these kinds of acts are common in these patients. Borderline personality disorder must be differentiated from depressive and bipolar disorder.

Avoidant personality disorder must be differentiated from anxiety disorders, especially social phobia. Dependent personality disorder must be differentiated from depression and anxiety disorders. Obsessive–compulsive personality disorder must be differentiated from obsessive–compulsive disorder and hoarding disorder.

All personality disorders must be differentiated from one another.

DIAGNOSTIC FALLACIES

Personality disorders are usually underdiagnosed rather than overdiagnosed. Many of these patients provide history of long-standing symptoms since early adulthood, but they are mistaken for other psychiatric disorders.

MANAGEMENT

Cognitive behaviour therapy with behavioural shaping is used for the management of personality disorders. Pharmacotherapy is equally important to control the symptoms, eg, aggression may be controlled using valproate (250–1000 mg/day), lithium (300–900mg/day) or antipsychotics (risperidone 2–12 mg/day) depending upon whether the aggression contains the affective component; is predatory or presented with or without abnormal EEG. Mood may be managed using mood stabilizers (valproate 250–1000 mg/day), selective serotonin reuptake inhibitors (sertraline 25–100 mg/day) or atypical antipsychotics (quetuapine 25–600 mg/day). For anxiety, benzodiazepines (clonazepam 0.25–2 mg/day) or low-dose atypical antipsychotics (risperidone 0.5 mg/day; olanzapine 2.5 mg/day) may be used. Psychotic symptoms may be controlled using antipsychotics.

COURSE AND PROGNOSIS

Personality disorders often follow a chronic and persistent course.

SUMMARY

- Personality disorders appear during late adolescence.
- They govern the behaviour in an enduring and pervasive manner.
- Their symptoms are often subtle and most of the patients do not get clinical attention.
- They are inherited but due to brain plasticity, environment also plays a role in their development.

FURTHER READING

1. American Psychiatric Association. (2013). "Diagnostic and Statistical Manual of Mental Disorders." 5th edit, Author, Washington, DC.
2. Sadock B. J., Sadock V. A., and Ruiz P. (2009). "Kaplan and Sadock's Comprehensive Textbook of Psychiatry." 9th edit, Lippincott Williams & Wilkins, Philadelphia, Pa, USA.
3. World Health Organization. (1992). "The ICD-10 Classification of Mental and Behavioural Disorders: Clinical Descriptions and Diagnostic Guidelines." Author, Geneva.

EATING DISORDERS

3.9

Ravi Gupta

Eating disorders are characterized by misperception of body image (feeling that one is excessively fat, whereas one is not) along with consequent change in the eating habits and food-related behaviour to bring oneself to (mis)perceived normal shape (Fig. 3.9.1). Gradually the sufferer accumulates medical/physiological complications associated with the change in food-related behaviour.

Hence, misperception of body image is the central factor to the development of eating disorders and other symptoms may be viewed as the result of this false perception. Depending upon the status of body weight, this disorder is differentiated into two subtypes—anorexia nervosa (where a person is not able to maintain normal weight compared to his/her ideal age and height-related weight) and bulimia nervosa (where a person either has not lost the weight or has gained the weight). These patients are often engaged in inappropriate behaviours to compensate for the weight gain, eg, excessive exercise, inducing vomiting and inappropriate use of laxatives and purgatives. These behaviours can lead to muscle damage, nutritional deficiency, dyselectrolytaemia and hormonal imbalances. Hence, they may present as medical emergencies.

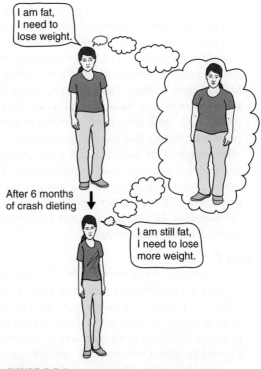

FIGURE 3.9.1

Body image misperception in eating disorders.

NOSOLOGY

DSM-5 and ICD-10 differ in the categories of eating disorders as mentioned in Table 3.9.1.

Table 3.9.1 Comparative Nosology of Eating Disorders	
DSM-5	**ICD-10**
Anorexia nervosa	Anorexia nervosa
Bulimia nervosa	Bulimia nervosa
Binge eating disorder	–

VIGNETTE

Case 1

A 17-year-old female was brought to the hospital because she fainted thrice in her classroom the previous day. Parents informed that she was engaged in 'strict' dieting since the past 6 months. She used to skip meals and whenever she was eating, the food was mostly of low calorie. She stopped eating any kind of food that contained even a small amount of fat, eg, milk, eggyolk, fried vegetables, icecreams, rice and canned juices. She was fond of sweets earlier but she had not eaten a single piece of sweet since the past 6 months. She was mostly surviving on salads (without any dressing) and water. On the insistence of her family, she would eat a *roti* (bread) with small amount of vegetable or *dal* (pulses) but would vomit it afterwards. The girl provided a history that she was getting fat, so she wanted to lose weight through dieting. She often exercised for more than 2 h a day and lost 15 kg in the past 2 months. Further interview revealed that she often used purgatives and often induced vomiting by putting finger into her mouth after having food. She had sunken eyes, dry skin, dry tongue and appeared cachexic. Her height was 154 cm and her weight was 32 kg. Her pulse was 104/min with blood pressure of 80/50 mmHg. Her conjunctiva was pale. Based on the history and examination, diagnosis of anorexia nervosa was made.

Case 2

A 22-year-old female was sent by the endocrinologist because she was gaining weight since the past 1 year. She had gained around 18 kg during this period. Endocrinological work-up did not contribute to her obesity. During interview she described periods when she felt a loss of control over the amount of food and ate larger portions than the usual. She expressed her concerns regarding putting on weight and was desperate to lost it. She sometimes exercised vigorously, sometimes induced vomiting and at other times used laxatives after episodes of uncontrolled eating. There was no history to suggest anorexia nervosa. Vital signs were within normal limits. Mental status examination disclosed distress, preoccupation with body weight and loss of control over eating. Based on the history and examination, diagnosis of bulimia nervosa was made.

CLINICAL PRESENTATION

Patients with anorexia nervosa often lack insight into their problem and hence almost never seek help themselves. They are unwilling for treatment, as they do not perceive their condition as pathological and often brought to the clinicians by the family members who are concerned about weight loss or medical complications of forced starvation. The symptoms must be present for at least 3 months before making the diagnosis. Basic problem is regarding misperceived body image where they perceive themselves fatter than they actually are. Along with this misperception, there is a morbid preoccupation for thinness and the sufferer keeps on thinking about means to lose weight or not to gain weight. These patients often lose weight and on examination their weight is below the normal of optimal weight for age, height and gender. This loss of weight is not able to solve their fear and they still fear of gaining weight. They appear ignorant to their weight loss or underweight status and still demand to lose some more weight.

Because of the fear of gaining weight, they try to minimize the amount of food or the calorie intake. To compensate their fear, they are often involved in one of the two methods—first, to restrict the amount of food intake by fasting or missing meals (restricting type anorexia nervosa),and second, they eat large amount of food in a single go and then either purge or vomit the food (binge eating/purging type anorexia nervosa). They induce vomit by putting their fingers in the mouth or use emetics. Some of them misuse laxatives or enemas to purge the food. Others go one step further and use diuretics to lose weight or may be engaged in heavy exercise to burn calories.

However, these persons rarely have anorexia *per se*. They appreciate their hunger but force themselves not to eat because of weight related issues. They may keep on collecting recipes or cook multicourse meals for other people. Many of them handle food in strange manners, like hiding it at inappropriate places. They may spend hours playing with food in peculiar ways. However, whenever somebody tries to bring this weird behaviour to their notice, they may become angry or simply deny doing that. Another important feature of anorexia nervosa is amenorrhoea for at least 3 months in absence of other known causes of amenorrhoea. It develops because of disturbance in the hypothlamo–pituitary–gonadal axis.

Contrary to anorexia nervosa, bulimia nervosa is characterized by recurrent episodes of binge eating which can be defined as eating larger portion as compared to usual amount, along with the feeling of lack of control over eating during that period. Patient may be engaged in recurrent behaviours to prevent weight gain. These behaviours must occur at least once a week for at least 3 months to qualify for the diagnosis of bulimia nervosa. However, binge eating should not occur during the period of anorexia nervosa.

Some persons have binge eating episodes without compensatory behaviours. This condition is termed as binge eating disorder.

Clinical examination shows signs of starvation and findings of compensatory behaviours. Hence, patients of anorexia nervosa are often underweight and skinny. They may develop lanugo hair all over the body. Those who induce vomiting by inserting finger in the mouth have callosities on the back of hands or on knuckles. Their denture may be damaged because of recurrent reflux of acid in the vomit. Their salivary glands may be enlarged. Vomiting induces hypokalemic alkalosis and its signs may be seen. Persons using purging or diuretic may present with dehydration, hyponatraemia, hypomagnesaemia, hypophosphetaemia. Hypotension may be present consequent to hyponatraemia and dehydration. ECG may show arrhythmia or bradycardia. Bone mineral density is often low with osteopoenia and osteoporosis. Hypercholesterolaemia may be noticed along with elevation of hepatic enzymes and serum amylase.

NEUROBIOLOGY

Although the environmental factors are important in the *expression* of eating disorders, these disorders cannot be ignored just as a learned behaviour. Many of the factors point towards the underlying biological factors, eg, the disorders run in families, concordance rates in monozygotic twins are higher than in dizygotic twins, symptoms are stereotyped across cultures and lastly, they appear at a certain age (adolescence). Most importantly, environmental pressures for 'thinness' are rampant, whereas eating disorders are seen only in a handful of individuals. Taken together, these factors suggest that disorder develop in an individual who is biologically predisposed (ie, born with the genes) and these genes become manifest when an appropriate environment becomes available. The environment includes physiological factors (availability of gonadal hormones at puberty which may be one reason why it appears during adolescence) or the learned behaviour (social pressure for maintaining weight or body shape—this is why it is more common in certain occupations). Still, exact pathophysiological mechanisms remain to be explored.

Normally, the signals for the taste of food reach to the nucleus tractus solitaries (NTS) and then relayed to thalamus. From thalamus they reach the primary gustatory cortex, which is located in the anterior insula and frontal operculum. From here, the signals are transmitted to the ventral striatum and amygdala that attach a 'reward' with the food. One stream then relays the signals to lateral hypothalamus (satiety) and to frontal cortex. Attachment of 'reward' to the food sets up or modifies the already present information in the frontal cortex and decides whether we like the food or not. In future, it also provides a hedonic value to the same food and helps us in making decision, whether we want to eat or not. Another stream from amygdala and ventral striatum relays the signals to ventral tegmental area (VTA) that sends dopaminergic signals to higher subcortical and cortical regions, thus completing the reward circuit (Fig. 3.9.2)

In eating disorders, this reward pathway is dysfunctional. Bulimia patients have reduced dopamine surge in striatum when exposed to food and reverse occurs in the anorexia nervosa (refer to 1 in Fig. 3.9.2). It must be noted that the frontal cortex has bilateral connections with amygdala to control its activity. Anorexia patients develop anxiety when exposed to food and thus, there is hyper activation of amygdala. Normally, frontal cortex inhibits amygdala's activity; however, in anorexia patients this white matter connection gets weaker; thus, hyperactivity persist

Pathways responsible for various symptoms of eating disorders

1. ↓ Reward, dysphoria, ↑ motor activity
2. ↓ Cortical control over amygdala
   (Food appears anxiety provoking)
3. Body image disturbance, not
   eating even when malnourished.
4. ↑ Activity- ↑ anxiety, specially related to food

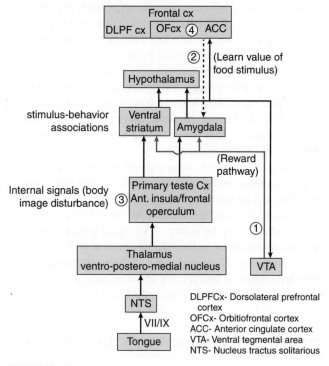

FIGURE 3.9.2

Neurobiology of eating disorders.

and they perceive food as a threat (2 in Fig. 3.9.2). Insula is responsible for the introceptive stimuli from the body. Thus, it helps us to determine the body shape, its energy needs and metabolic status. A dysfunction in this region has been proposed to be associated with bodyimage disturbance that is observed in these patients (but not in binge eating disorder (BED) patients; refer to 3 in Fig. 3.9.2). Moreover, these patients have higher anxiety owing to higher activity of orbitofrontal cortex and anterior cingulate gyrus; thus, a variety of anxious behaviours are seen in these patients (please refer to 4 in Fig. 3.9.2).

EPIDEMIOLOGY AND RISK FACTORS

Anorexia nervosa has a prevalence of 0.4% in adolescent girls and the disorder usually starts during adolescence. Females are nearly 10 times more likely to develop the disorders as compared to males. Bulimia nervosa has the prevalence of 1–5%, whereas binge eating disorder is seen in 0.8% men and 1.6% women. Positive family history increases the risk of all these disorders.

DIFFERENCES BETWEEN ICD-10 AND DSM-5

ICD-10 has some differences in the symptomatology from DSM-5. These are depicted in Table 3.9.2.

Table 3.9.2 Differences in Symptoms in ICD-10 from DSM-5

	Anorexia Nervosa	Bulimia Nervosa
Body weight	Weight 15% below the expected weight	None

DIFFERENTIAL DIAGNOSIS

Medical causes of weight loss: Hyperthyroidism, diabetes, chronic infections, myopathies and carcinomas.

Depression: Depressed persons are often not concerned with their body image, rather they lose appetite. In contrast, persons with anorexia nervosa have normal appetite and feel hungry but voluntarily restrict calorie intake for weight related issues. Depressed person lose interest in almost everything and do not collect recipes or prepare food like anorexia nervosa patients.

Bulimia nervosa: Both anorexia nervosa and bulimia nervosa may present with binge eating episodes. But bulimic patients rarely lose weight. In addition, binge eating episodes are usually egodystonic and they seek help because of this reason.

Body dysmorphic disorder: Symptoms are limited to one or the other organ of the body; these patients are not preoccupied with their weight.

Klein Levin syndrome (KLS): Bulimia nervosa and binge eating disorder should be differentiated from KLS.KLS is characterized by episodes of hypersomnia. This may be idiopathic or secondary. This also starts during adolescence but more common in boys.

Kluver–Bucy syndrome: Characterized by visual agnosia, hyperorality (every object is examined by licking or biting), hypersexuality and hyperphagia.

DIAGNOSTIC FALLACIES

Paranoid schizophrenia: These patients are not concerned with the caloric value and weight gaining properties of food; rather they avoid food because they think that it is poisoned.

Atypical depression: Depression is characterized by hypersexuality, hypersomnolence and hyperphagia in addition to depression.

Sleep-related eating disorder: This is a parasomnia in which person binge eats during period of sleep. However, person is often oblivious of his act the next day.

Night eating syndrome: Characterized by episodes of eating during the night. However, the person is awake and alert during these episodes.

Voluntary fasting: Voluntary fasting for prolonged periods, either religious or as a mark of passive aggression, should not be mistaken for eating disorders.

MANAGEMENT

Mainstay of management is cognitive behaviour therapy (CBT) where dysfunctional beliefs are challenged and substituted. Patients are trained to identify their maladaptive behaviours like restriction, purging or vomiting and to stop them. They are advised to improve and monitor their food intake. Their food-related emotions and feelings are also addressed. Pharmacotherapy is required to address comorbidities. Antidepressants may help to curtail depression and anxiety disorders. Choice of antidepressant depends upon the comorbid conditions and target symptoms. However, selective serotonin reuptake inhibitors, eg, escitalopram (5–20 mg/day) have been found effective. In extreme cases, hospitalization is mandatory for anyone who presents with medical complications. They are offered supportive treatment and nutritional replacement. However, this should be done in consultation with a physician and a dietician as food ingestion after prolonged fasting makes them prone to develop refeeding syndrome.

COURSE AND PROGNOSIS

Prognoses are poor in anorexia nervosa and only 25% patients achieve complete remission. Adequate treatment at the outset is necessary to improve the chances of remission. If adequate treatment is not given, the disease may take a chronic course. This negatively affects the quality of life and the patient may be a burden with recurrent hospitalizations. Bulimia nervosa also has the relapsing and remitting course with multiple episodes in the lifetime. Binge eating disorder usually follows the same course. A sizeable number of patients may sometimes commit suicide and, hence, they must be screened for suicidal thoughts.

SUMMARY

- Eating disorders are characterized by body image misperception.
- These disorders have neurobiological underpinnings.
- These patients often present in the emergency with complications.

FURTHER READING

1. American Psychiatric Association. (2013). "Diagnostic and Statistical Manual of Mental Disorders." 5th edit, Author, Washington, DC.
2. Frank G. K. W. (2013). Altered Brain Reward Circuits in Eating Disorders: Chicken or the Egg? *Current Psychiatry Report*, 15:396.
3. World Health Organization. (1992). "The ICD-10 Classification of Mental and Behavioural Disorders: Clinical Descriptions and Diagnostic Guidelines." Author, Geneva.

SOMATIC SYMPTOMS AND RELATED DISORDERS

3.10

Ravi Gupta

This group includes those disorders where patients present with persistent preoccupation with somatic symptoms. These symptoms may occur in the presence of known medical disorders, but in such settings the concern is excessive as compared to underlying pathology and cause significant distress and concern. In some cases, the symptoms may not be explained by any of the known medical disorders. However, mere absence of medical explanation does not imply the psychological nature of the symptoms, rather communicates that either we do not have adequate knowledge to explain the pathophysiology (we are dealing with a yet to be described disorder or syndrome) or that the pathology lies at the central level, ie, brain.

You must understand that the entire body has its representation in the brain. Sensory information from whole body, including one from viscera, reaches the brain through the connection between peripheral nervous system and central nervous system. Thus, in these disorders, brain areas dealing with the interoceptive information become dysfunctional.

NOSOLOGY

There is some difference between the nomenclature provided by DSM-5 and ICD-10 (Table 3.10.1).

Table 3.10.1 Comparative Nosology of Somatic Symptoms Disorders	
DSM-5	**ICD-10**
Somatic symptoms disorder	Somatization disorder
Illness anxiety disorder	Hypochondriacal disorder
Conversion disorder (functional neurological symptom disorder)	Dissociative disorder
Factitious disorder	Intentional production or feigning of symptoms or disabilities, either physical or psychological (factitious disorder)

VIGNETTE

A 30-year-old man presented with complaints of pain in the body for the past 6 months. He describes it as both arthralgia and myalgia that limits his working efficiency. He also complains of headache of unspecified type, problems in digestion, episodes of diarrhoea and constipation lasting for few days, occasional palpitations, memory lapses, poor appetite and pain in the abdomen. He also feels burning sensation while voiding. Most of the time, he remains concerned with these symptoms and has undergone multiple investigations, none of which showed a significant abnormality. He is a known case of acid peptic disease and bronchial asthma. He is taking treatment for the same. Physical examination shows that vital signs were within normal limits. Mental status examination disclosed distress and preoccupation with the body symptoms. Based on the history and clinical examination, diagnosis of somatic symptoms disorder was made.

CLINICAL PICTURE

Patients with these disorders have excessive concerns for the somatic symptoms, clearly in excess to the underlying pathology. These symptoms may be episodic, recurrent or chronic in nature. However, in patients with chronic disorder, these symptoms may have episodic exacerbation. These patients often undergo multiple investigations that do not demonstrate significant pathology. However, it must be understood that sensitivity towards pain vary from person to person and what appears as an insignificant pain to one may be severe for the other. These people often perceive normal body symptoms, eg, pulsation of abdominal aorta, abdominal sounds, physiological hyperpnoea or palpitations occurring in setting of exertion as abnormal. When they are explained regarding physiological nature of these types of symptoms, they are not able to accept it and may change the consulting physician.

Presence of known medical disorder does not rule out the somatic symptoms disorder and absence of medical explanation does not lead to diagnosis of somatic symptoms disorder. In a fair number of individuals, they are present with medical disorders. These symptoms often take the central role in the life of these patients and they are quite distressed about them.

Patients with functional neurological symptoms disorder may present with nonepileptic seizures, monoplegia, paraplegia, hemiplegia, sensory loss, mutism (not aphasia), seizures, etc. Their focus is the presence of somatic symptoms that they want to get treated. Loss of sensation in these patients often defies the dermatomal distribution of nerves and is usually strictly along one line (see below).

Patients with factitious disorder often produce the symptoms without any apparent motive (otherwise it would be termed malingering). They often seek treatment repeatedly (like other patients in this group of disorders). They may inflict injury upon themselves or may consume substances that can produce symptoms. They remain focused on the somatic symptoms and require repeated reassurance and treatment for their symptoms.

Comparison of symptoms of various disorders is depicted in Table 3.10.2.

Table 3.10. 2 Tabular Comparison of Different Disorders

	Somatic Symptoms Disorder	Illness Anxiety Disorder	Functional Neuro-logical Symptoms Disorder	Factitious Disorder
Presenting symptoms	Excessive concern with the bodily symptoms with or without presence of medical disorder In the 'persistent pain type', patients present with pre-dominant complaints of pain	Fixation with having a medical illness with high level of anxiety regarding health. The engage-ment in getting their body checked up or undergoing investiga-tions is excessive	Symptoms suggest-ing sensory, motor, cognitive, emotional or autonomic distur-bance, eg, hemiple-gia, sensory loss, paresthesia, mutism, seizures La belle indifference, secondary gain and presence of trauma are *not* essential for diagnosis.	Patients falsify the presence of symp-toms or disease and may even consume substances or inflict injury to appear diseased. When the preexisting disease is present, they may do necessary acts to increase its severity. When the disorder is 'imposed on another', the patient does the acts necessary to produce symptoms in another person. However, they do not have any apparent motivation to do the same
Duration	6 months required for persistent somatic symptom disorder(SSD)	Symptoms must be present for 6 months	If more than 6 months, considered persistent	Not required
Nature of illness	Persistent symptoms	Persistent symptoms	Episodic nature	Transient or persis-tent
Age of onset	Adulthood but may be seen in children	Adulthood	Adolescence	Early adulthood
Prevalence	Not known; F > M	Not known	Not known	Not known

NEUROBIOLOGY

We have limited understanding of the neurobiology of somatic symptoms disorders. Here, we are describing the neurobiology with reference to the pain, although similar pathology may be implicated in the motor, autonomic or any other symptom seen in somatic symptoms disorder.

Fundamental to the neurobiology of these disorders are the facts that (1) pain has both sensory and emotional component (localized in sensory cortex and cingulate cortex, respectively); (2) stress-led hypothalamo-pituitary- adrenal (HPA) axis activation produce immunological effects by increasing pro-inflammatory cytokines; and (3) neural areas that modulate distress overlap with those involved in processing of the pain.

Areas that are involved in somatosensory processing (eg, insula and thalamus) and areas that deal with emotional issues (eg, limbic lobes, anterior cingulate gyrus and amygdala) are over active in these patients both at rest and also after application of mild stimulus. This is why these patients get emotionally disrupted even with mild stimulus.

Abnormal sensory gating of the afferent impulses makes them highly sensitive towards the stimuli coming from internal and peripheral organs. Thus, these patients perceive a mild stimulus in an exaggerated manner, eg, mild pain as severe, mild distension of viscera as one beyond the limit of tolerance. Top-down gating of the sensory stimuli, especially to that of pain, is less pronounced in these patients leading to increased perception of pain. When the sensitization occurs at the level of brain, variety of symptoms develops depending upon the area involved. When the sensitization involves A-beta type nerve fibres, which normally carry pain and touch sensations, allodynia is seen (nonpainful stimulus is painful); when it involves A-delta type nerve fibres that carry pain associated with thermal or chemical sensation or type C-nerve fibres that carry pain, hyperalgesia appears. This could be associated with dysfunction in the descending serotonergic and opioidergic pathways (Fig. 3.10.1).

Stress is able to invoke the inflammatory markers in the body (please refer to Chapter 3.6 on stress and related disorders). Whereas acute stress usually has an immunosuppressive effect, chronic stress increases the concentration of pro-inflammatory markers in the body, including IL-1, IL-6 and TNF-α. These cytokines can alter the homoeostasis by exerting paracrine actions. One of the actions of these

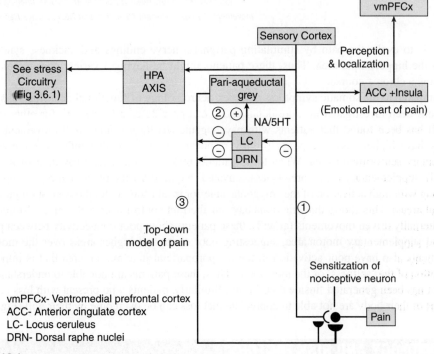

FIGURE 3.10.1

Neurobiological mechanisms underlying somatic symptoms disorder.

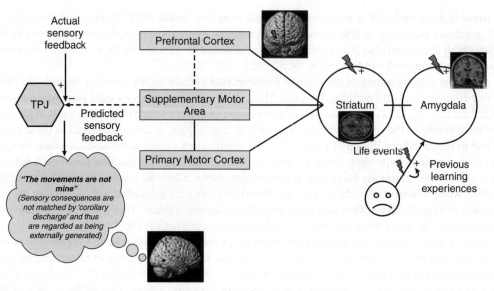

FIGURE 3.10.2

Neurobiology of psychogenic movement disorder. TPJ-Temporo-parietal junction.

(Source: *Mehta AR, Rowe JE, Schrag AE (2013). Imaging Psychogenic movement Disorders. Current Neurology and Neuroscience Report, 13:402).*

cytokines is to evoke the pain by stimulating peripheral nerve endings and 'sickness syndrome' by acting on the hippocampal area. Thus, these patients might be having a variety of symptoms, which often follow a chronic course.

As compared to the somatic symptoms disorder, neurobiology of functional neurological symptoms disorder has been investigated in more detail and it can provide us a framework for other symptoms as well. It has been found that patients with psychogenic (*really psychogenic?*) movement disorders inherently have higher startle response (highly responsive amygdala) that influences the activity of supplementary sensorimotor area. When these patients make any movement (by their own will or on command), supplementary motor area is less activated (required for the planning/preparation of movement) along with high activation of the amygdala, anterior insula and bilateral posterior cingulate cortex (emotional areas). This shows that emotions have an aberrant control over motor areas. Moreover, during the internally driven movements (at will), these patients show poor connectivity between prefrontal cortex and supplementary motor area, suggesting poor control of higher areas over the motor areas. These patients also have poor activation in the temporoparietal junction, an area that is important for the prediction of the 'selfness' of the movement. Thus, these patients are not able to understand that the movement has been generated 'inside their brain'. Similarly, patients who present with loss of function of any part of their body are not able to appreciate that loss can be overcome by their will (Fig. 3.10.2).

EPIDEMIOLOGY AND RISK FACTORS

Prevalence of these disorders is not known. However, they appear to be more common among females. Risk factors are not known though life stressors have been implicated in development of these disorders.

DIFFERENCE IN ICD-10 FROM DSM-5

Description of symptoms in ICD-10 is different from DSM-5. This is depicted in Table 3.10.3.

DIFFERENTIAL DIAGNOSIS

These disorders should be differentiated form autoimmune disorders that affect visceral parts as well as the masculoskeletal framework.

These disorders must be differentiated from fibromyalgia and chronic fatigue syndrome. Fibromyalgia is diagnosed when the patient has pain above and below the waist, on both sides of the body and has at least 13 tender points out of 18. Whether it represents the somatic symptom disorder remains to be defined. Chronic fatigue syndrome is characterized by 'remains always fatigued' or 'easily gets fatigued' and complaints last for more than 6 months.

They should be differentiated from each other, as discussed in the chapter.

They must be differentiated from substance withdrawal, particularly, opioid withdrawal.

Malingering presents with 'intentional' feigning of symptoms for an apparent motive, eg, missing the examination and for avoiding any responsibility. However, in these disorders, motive is not apparent.

Functional neurological symptom disorder can be differentiated from mimicking disorders by following:

- Patients with seizures may have an aura, short lasting episodes of convulsions, post-ictal delirium, loss of consciousness, involuntary micturition and defecation and tongue bite during the episode of generalized tonic-clonic seizure. These features are absent in nonepileptic seizures. These episodes are often stereotyped in contrary to what is seen during nonepileptic seizures. Physical examination reveals extensor planters and sluggish deep tendon reflexes after true seizures. Intra-ictal EEG is most significant in differentiating between the two.
- Sensory loss often follows anatomical boundaries rather than dermatomal distribution, eg, there may be a strict demarcation at wrist, ankle or any other joint between the areas of absence and presence of sensation. Similar strict midline demarcation is reported when the sensory loss involves scalp, face, chest, abdomen and back (Fig. 3.10.3).

Table 3.10.3 Differences in ICD-10 from DSM-5

Somatic Symptoms Disorder	Illness Anxiety Disorder	Somatic Symptoms Disorder: Persistent Pain Type
2 years duration Repeated consultation means three or more consultations	6 months duration of symptoms	Persistent pain for at least 6 months
Symptoms must be present from at least two of the following groups—gastrointestinal system; cardiovascular system; genitourinary system; skin and pain symptoms	Two or more diseases of which at least one should be named by the patient Presumed deformity of the body (includes body dysmorphic disorder)	

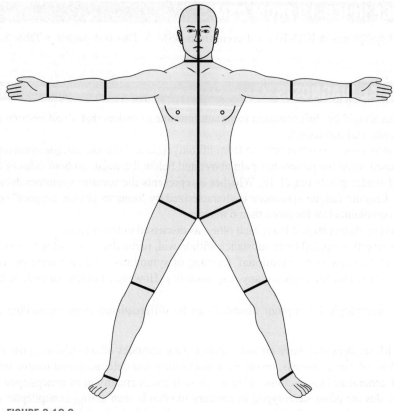

FIGURE 3.10.3

Symptoms boundaries in conversion disorders.

- Vision loss is often in the form of tunnel vision.
- Hoover sign can be used to differentiate the alleged weakness in lower limbs from true paresis. Normally, when one leg is raised against gravity or resistance, the contra-lateral leg extends. To test it, a patient is asked to lie down. Then the examiner places his hand below the heel of normal leg and asks the patient to raise the paralyzed leg, but keeping it straight. In case of true paresis, patient will make an effort to flex the paralyzed limb and the you will feel the pressure on the hand, kept below normal heel.

DIAGNOSTIC FALLACIES

Simple partial seizures may be mistaken for functional neurological symptoms disorders, especially those arising from deeper brain structures. Scalp EEG is able to pick only the cortical activity and thus seizures arising from insula, deep nuclei, hippocampus and mesial temporal lobe may be missed.

Somatic symptoms are very common in patients with sleep disorders, especially those leading to nonrefreshing sleep, eg, insomnia, restless legs syndrome and sleep apnoea. A clinician not having the adequate knowledge of sleep disorders may keep their focus on somatic symptoms disorders, without addressing the underlying cause.

MANAGEMENT

Nonpharmacological management is an important aspect and it consists of reassurance, relaxation and cognitive behaviour therapy. Whereas relaxation therapies help in just relieving the anxiety, reassurance helps to build the confidence. However, false reassurance should be avoided considering the chronic course of the illness. Cognitive behaviour therapy aims at identifying the dysfunctional beliefs and correcting them.

Pharmacotherapy consists of antidepressants, particularly drugs from the selective serotonin reuptake inhibitor (SSRI) and selective serotonin and noradrenaline reuptake inhibitors (SNRIs). Fluoxetine (20–60 mg/day), paroxetine (12.5–37.5 mg/day), duloxetine (20–40 mg/day) or venlafaxine (37.5–225 mg/day) may be tried. Anxiolytics (clonazepam 0.25–2 mg/day) may be used as an adjuvant therapy.

COURSE AND PROGNOSIS

These disorders often run a chronic course with relapses and remissions. Some of these, eg, conversion disorder, can have acute symptoms with short-lasting episodes with complete interepisodic recovery.

SUMMARY

- Somatic symptoms disorder and conversion disorder have a neurobiological basis.
- These disorders are common and frequently poorly treated.
- These disorders often run a chronic course.
- Adequate treatment can improve the condition and quality of life.

FURTHER READING

1. American Psychiatric Association. (2013). "Diagnostic and Statistical Manual of Mental Disorders." 5th edit, Author, Washington, DC.
2. Dimsdale J. E., and Dantzer R. (2007). A Biological Substrate for Somatoform Disorders: Importance of Pathophysiology. *Psychosomatic Medicine*, 69:850–854.
3. Kim S. E., and Chang L. (2012). Overlap Between Functional GI Disorders and Other Functional Syndromes: What Are the Underlying Mechanisms? *Neurogastroenterology& Motility*, 24.doi:10.1111/j.1365-2982.2012.01993.x.
4. Landa A., Peterson B. S., and Fallon B. A. (2012). Somatoform Pain: A Developmental Theory and Translational Research Review. *Psychosomatic Medicine*, 74:717–727.
5. Mehta A. R., Rowe J. E., and Schrag A. E. (2013). Imaging Psychogenic Movement Disorders. *Current Neurology and Neuroscience Report*, 13:402.
6. World Health Organization. (1992). "The ICD-10 Classification of Mental and Behavioural Disorders: Clinical Descriptions and Diagnostic Guidelines." Author, Geneva.

DISSOCIATIVE DISORDERS 3.11

Ravi Gupta

Dissociative disorders are those conditions where all mental faculties, eg, consciousness, awareness, memory, identity, perception, emotions and behaviour, get interrupted and the person has a gap or alteration in their continuity.

Normally, all of us are aware of the surroundings and are able to integrate all the perceptions with our emotions and behave accordingly. However, in these conditions, this integration, which is normal and required for daily functioning, becomes fragmented. Thus, these patients report a gap in their memory, experience a change in their personality or feel some unusual experiences, eg, out-of-body incidents. These symptoms usually emerge in a highly emotional environment, eg, after a significant trauma or stress.

NOSOLOGY

There are some differences in the nomenclature of these disorders between DSM-5 and ICD-10 (Table 3.11.1).

VIGNETTE

A 35-year-old man was brought with complaints of significant memory loss. This memory loss started 30 days back, when he lost his wife. Since then, he is not able to recognize family members from his wife's side and his children. He lost his wife in a car accident but, fortunately, he did not suffer any injury. People around him reported that he was transiently unconscious for few minutes. His neuroimaging (MRI of the brain) did not reveal any injury. He is now not able to recall the car accident, and also not able to provide information where they were heading to and other details related to that travel. Physical examination reveals that vital parameters are within normal limits. Mental status examination discloses a gap in the memory that is limited to his children and relatives of wife's side. Based on the history and examination, diagnosis of dissociative amnesia was made.

CLINICAL PICTURE

Dissociative amnesia is characterized by a significant gap in the recall of memories that are otherwise resistant to any kind of damage, eg., autobiographical memories (Who am I? Who are my family members? What do I do?) or episodic memories (What did I do in the past 7 days? Did any significant event occur during the past 10 days that was related to me?). Some of these patients have partial and episodic recall of the events that occurred during the symptomatic period.

Table 3.11.1 Comparative Nosology of Dissociative Disorders

DSM-5	ICD-10
Dissociative identity disorder	Multiple personality disorder
Dissociative amnesia	Dissociative amnesia
Depersonalization/ derealization disorder	–

In dissociative identity disorder, patient may assume one or more personalities during the symptomatic period that may last for some time. Each of these personalities has a different kind of behaviour, feelings and emotions that is clearly deviant from the patient's own personality. All the events that happened during personality "A" may not be recalled when it ceases to exist and the patient assumes a new personality e.g., personality "B". These patients often find some objects in their bags for which they have no memory where did they get them or do some acts which they may not recall when they have another personality (they may have bought it or committed it during personality A, but unable to recall when they are in personality B).

Some patients may complain that the environment that they live in appears unreal to them, as if they are living in a fantasy world and they feel detached from the environment (derealization). At other times, they may have out-of-body experiences that they are watching their body objectively while they are floating in the air (depersonalization).

Comparison of the symptomatology of these disorders is depicted in Table 3.11.2.

Table 3.11.2 Comparison of Clinical Picture of Different Disorders

	Dissociative Identity Disorder	Dissociative Amnesia	Depersonalization/Derealization Disorder
Symptoms	Assumption of a new personality and the patient may fluctuate between two or more personalities. There is a discontinuity in the emotions, behaviour, memory of one personality that is usually not accessible to other.	Patients are unable to recall important biographical memories, especially those which are traumatic in nature.	Feel that they have detached from their 'self' (depersonalization) that includes emotions, sensations and thoughts (I have emotions but I am not able to appreciate them/I have thoughts but I do not feel that they are my own/I know you touching me but not able to acknowledge it). People with derealization feel as if they are living in an imaginary world with intact reality testing.
Discontinuity	A gap in the personality.	A gap occurs in the memories for the period of amnesia.	Discontinuity in the feeling of reality and continuity between self and one's own psyche or the environment.
Duration	Not specified	Not specified	Not specified

NEUROBIOLOGY

Neurobiology of dissociative disorders is not well understood. The evidence links pathology between the limbic lobe and the temporal lobe; however, these findings have emerged out of the epilepsy and migraine patients. Pharmacological evidence gathered from the cannabis and ketamine users has suggested that this could be mediated by the diminished activity of glutaminergic-NMDA receptors that are found in abundance in amygdala, hippocampus and cortical areas. Depersonalization that is seen after lysergide (LSD) and psilocybine, points to the involvement of serotonergic system in the pathogenesis of these disorders. However, further data is not available as of now.

EPIDEMIOLOGY AND RISK FACTORS

Prevalence of these disorders is between 1% and 2% in the United States with equal gender proportions. Transient episodes of depersonalization and derealization are more common and most of the people have experienced them at least once in their life.

DIFFERENCE BETWEEN ICD-10 AND DSM-5

There are some differences in the symptomatology between ICD-10 and DSM-5. These are shown in Table 3.11.3.

DIFFERENTIAL DIAGNOSIS

These disorders must be differentiated from one another. They must be differentiated from post-traumatic stress disorder which also has other symptoms, eg, flashbacks or sympathetic arousal.

They must be differentiated from seizure disorders, particularly temporal lobe seizures that may appear with similar symptoms since these mental faculties are regulated by temporal lobe.

They must be differentiated from functional neurological symptoms disorder, particularly nonepileptic convulsions where amnesia may be reported for the event.

Symptoms arising because of substance intoxication, use disorder or withdrawal must be differentiated from these disorders.

Table 3.11.3 Differences in ICD-10 from DSM-5		
Dissociative Identity Disorder	**Dissociative Amnesia**	**Depersonalization/Derealization**
Stressor is required before the onset of symptom	Stressor is required before the onset of symptom	–

DIAGNOSTIC FALLACIES

Absence seizures may present with gaps in the memory, which should not be mistaken for dissociative amnesia. However, in the case of absence seizures, memory gap encompasses all kinds of memory and not just of one kind.

Complex partial seizures may lead to the temporary change in personality, which can be confused with dissociative identity disorder.

MANAGEMENT

There is no pharmacotherapy for dissociative amnesia. In some cases, cognitive therapy or hypnosis may be useful. Depersonalization and derealization are refractory to the treatment. As of now, we do not have any active intervention towards this; however, they should not be given relaxation therapy as it may precipitate the dissociative experience. Antidepressants may be tried for these disorders. An external sensory stimulus just at the start of these symptoms, eg, pinching may be helpful in terminating the episode. Antidepressants and anxiolytics may be tried in dissociative identity disorder.

COURSE AND PROGNOSIS

These disorders may be seen across all ages. Depersonalization and derealization may run a persistent course.

SUMMARY

- Dissociative disorders are prevalent. They are often mistaken for other psychiatric and neurological disorders.
- The key feature is an alteration in consciousness, awareness, memory or emotions that is usually transient.

FURTHER READING

1. American Psychiatric Association. (2013). "Diagnostic and Statistical Manual of Mental Disorders." 5th edit, Author, Washington, DC.
2. Simeon D. (2004). Depersonalization Disorder: A Contemporary Overview. *CNS Drugs*, 18:343–354.
3. World Health Organization. (1992). "The ICD-10 Classification of Mental and Behavioural Disorders: Clinical Descriptions and Diagnostic Guidelines." Author, Geneva.

SUBSTANCE-RELATED DISORDERS (ADDICTION)

4.1

Ravi Gupta

Addiction refers to a recurrent consumption of those substances that have an addiction potential by virtue of their ability to alter the higher mental functions and emotional state of a person. Many of the adolescents consume the substances of abuse out of their curiosity or under peer pressure (known as experimentation); however, only a few of them get addicted to it. Clinically, it translates to the disease model of addiction and is related to the problems in reward pathways of the brain. Based on the frequency, amount and compulsion to consume the substance, a patient may present with a variety of clinical syndromes, eg, intoxication, dependence or withdrawal, as we will discuss subsequently.

There are a number of substances; some stimulate the brain, whereas others depress neurological functions. Interestingly, different people have 'addiction' for different substances; some people consume more than one substance, but given a choice, they would prefer one given substance to others. Thus, individuals usually have a preference for one substance. This preference is thought to be associated with the effects of a given substance on the brain areas beyond the reward pathways.

Before proceeding further, it is important to understand the difference between intoxication, dependence and withdrawal; you must also be aware of the molecular biology of each of these entities. In this chapter, we will discuss about the neurobiology of addiction, we will discuss in brief the clinical presentation of common substances and management of respective conditions.

NOSOLOGY

DSM-5 and ICD-10 differ with respect to the terminologies used in addiction; this is presented in Table 4.1.1.

Table 4.1.1 Comparative Nosology of Substance Use Disorders

DSM-5	ICD-10
–	Harmful use
Intoxication	Intoxication
Use disorder	Dependence
Withdrawal	–

VIGNETTES

Case 1

A 30-year-old man presents to you with the complaints of 'feeling nervous' since 3 days. He is working in a multinational company and has recently felt 'extra pressure' of the work beyond his coping ability. There is a history of smoking five to seven cigarettes per day since 5 years. He says that this smoking increases during the stressful periods, but there have been periods lasting 3–4 months when he quit it without any problem. He knows that smoking is injurious but cannot quit because he considers that it helps to reduce the 'stress'. Physical examination does not reveal any abnormality. Based on the history and examination, diagnosis of nicotine use disorder was made.

Case 2

A 50-year-old man was brought to the emergency room in the state of altered consciousness. There is a history of consumption of alcohol (nearly seven to eight drinks) few hours back along with his friends. On examination, his gait was ataxic, speech was slurred and was delirious. His deep tendon reflexes were sluggish with a normal muscle tone.His relatives revealed that he was consuming alcohol for around 20 years. He started with one to two occasional (never more than two to three times a month) drinks initially, that too at social gatherings. Gradually, his frequency and quantity started increasing and, now, for around 10 years, he had been drinking approximately 8–10 pegs each day. He had communicated to his wife that lesser than this amount of alcohol did not provide him the 'kick' anymore. He had faced some problems at his work place due to daytime drinking and had also developed medical complications. However, he was not able to quit it because periods of abstinence were characterized by anxiety, tremulousness, craving for alcohol and poor concentration. Based on the history and clinical examination, diagnosis of alcohol use disorder with alcohol intoxication was made.

CLINICAL PICTURE

Clinical picture depends upon the type of substance that a person is consuming and the state of addiction, ie, use disorder, intoxication or withdrawal. These symptoms and signs are determined by the receptors in the brain on which they act. During intoxication, symptoms are determined by the action of substance on the neuronal receptors as well as peripheral organs. It develops after few hours of ingestion of substance in a large amount.

During use disorder, we see continued use of substance despite knowing that it is harmful for the personal, social and occupational functioning, craving (intense urge to consume the substance due to central effect), tolerance (increased amount of substance is required to produce same effect), withdrawal when the person does not consume the substance (symptoms opposite to acute effects of the substance) and excessive amount of time spent in seeking the substance (behavioural manifestation) along with peripheral effects of the substance.

Withdrawal occurs when a substance has been discontinued after consuming it in large amounts for a long time. Timing of appearance of withdrawal symptoms depends upon the half-life of the substance in question, how long was it consumed before cessation, its amount and the activity on the receptor. With substances of short half-life, these symptoms appear after few hours to few days; however, with long-acting substances, they may not appear at all, or may be subtle in presentation and limited to behavioural manifestations. Symptoms are also severe if the substance is pure agonist to its receptors and these receptors modulate the brain areas that have peripheral actions; eg, cannabis withdrawal does not have peripheral or somatic manifestations, whereas alcohol withdrawal has somatic manifestations in the form of tremors and seizures. Symptoms may be mild if the dose of the substance in question has been tapered before final cessation.

In this chapter, we will focus on commonly used substances—tobacco, alcohol, benzodiazepines, cannabis, inhalant and opioids; although there are a number of other substances that are consumed, eg, stimulants such as cocaine, methylphenidate and amphetamines; and hallucinogens such as phencyclidine and ketamine. A brief note will be mentioned about non-substance-related addiction, eg, gambling disorder.

To understand the clinical features, one must have knowledge regarding the receptors that the substances act on, their location in the brain and their actions. These are mentioned below.

NEUROBIOLOGICAL BASIS OF CLINICAL PRESENTATION OF INDIVIDUAL SUBSTANCES

TOBACCO

Tobacco is perhaps the most commonly consumed substance. It can be either chewed or can be smoked. However, in some parts of the globe including India, it is consumed by other methods, eg, sniffing, applying on gums and rinsing of mouth with tobacco water. It acts on the nicotinic cholinergic receptors that are present in various areas of the brain. In the hippocampus and 'diagonal band of Broca', these receptors help in memory formation. They are also seen in the ventral tegmental area (VTA) where they increase the release of dopamine in amygdala and nucleus accumbens, to provide a feeling of reward. Prefrontal cortical receptors stimulate this release further via acting on the glutaminergic receptors (see the pathways in Chapter 3.2 on schizophrenia) and locally also improve attention and concentration. Refer to Table 4.1.2 for clinical picture of tobacco addiction.

ALCOHOL

Alcohol acts on GABA receptors. These receptors are present diffusely in various brain areas, eg, cortex, amygdala and cerebellum. These areas govern most of the symptoms of alcohol addiction.

Table 4.1.2 Clinical Picture of Tobacco Addiction

Intoxication	Withdrawal	Use Disorder
Not known	Irritability, insomnia, dysphoria, restless, poor concentration, enhanced appetite	All features as mentioned in use disorder (see text);other symptoms include peripheral effects, eg, oral submucosal fibrosis, methaemoglobinaemia (in smokers due to CO inhalation), COPD, hypertension

Sedatives and hypnotics also act on these receptors and thus they have a similar picture. This is one reason why hypnotics are important in management of alcohol withdrawal (Table 4.1.3).

CANNABIS

Cannabis is another commonly abused substance in India. It is acquired from a plant *Cannabis sativa*. It can be used in many forms—green leaves are chewed (bhang), dried leaves can be smoked (ganja) or its resin can also be smoked (charas or hasish).

The active compound is Δ^9-tetra-hydrocannabinol (THC). It acts on cannabinoid receptors—CB1 receptors that are present in hippocampus, cerebrum, cerebellum, basal ganglia, thalamus, hypothalamus, amygdala and periaqueductal grey. See Table 4.1.4 for clinical picture of cannabis addiction.

INHALANTS

Some of the commonly used substances are glue, paint, thinner, nailpolish remover, petroleum products, various balms available in market for common cold and muscle sprains. It has been found that they act via NMDA receptors, GABA receptors, glycine receptors and 5-HT3 receptors. They also increase the dopamine in nucleus accumbens. Refer Table 4.1.5 for clinical picture of inhalant addiction.

Table 4.1.3. Clinical Picture of Alcohol Addiction

Intoxication	Withdrawal	Use-Disorder
Personality changes, eg, aggression, judgment errors, mood changes Slurred speech, ataxia, nystagmus, memory impairment, stupor, coma	Delirium, tremors, seizures, insomnia, vomiting, anxiety, visual hallucinations, sympathetic stimulation, agitation Usually develops after 4–12 h of abstinence from alcohol	All symptoms as mentioned in use disorder (see text);other features include hepatic compromise, dyslipidaemia, symptoms of vitamin B12 and thiamine deficiency, peripheral neuropathy, hypertension, pancreatitis

Table 4.1.4 Clinical Picture of Cannabis Addiction

Intoxication	Withdrawal	Use disorder
Behavioural changes, eg, euphoria, restlessness, depersonalization feeling, feeling of slowed time, conjunctival injection, dryness of mouth, increased heart rate and increased appetite	Agitation, anxiety, disturbed sleep, bad dreams, poor appetite, dysphoria, fever, abdominal pain, headache, tremors Usually develops within 1 week of abstinence from cannabis	All symptoms as mentioned in use disorder (see text);other features include conjunctival congestion, those smoking joints may have pulmonary complications of smoking

Table 4.1.5. Clinical Picture of Inhalant Addiction

Intoxication	Withdrawal	Use Disorder
A variety of symptoms may present and depend upon the substance in use, including dizziness, ataxia, slurring of speech, nystagmus, tremors, muscle weakness, diplopia, fatigue, coordination problems, mood changes	Not known	All symptoms as mentioned in 'use disorder' (see text);other features include finding the inhalants from the possession of patient, smell of substance from hands or clothes, rashes around mouth or nares

OPIOIDS AND OPIATES

Naturally acquired substances from the poppy plant are called opiates, whereas their synthetic derivatives are called opioids. Opiates are acquired from the flower of the poppy plant and can be consumed in different ways. Opium (*afeem or amal*) is the resin that is obtained after making a knick to the flower base. After the opium is obtained, leftover flower bases still contain small amount of opium and they are known as *doda or poste*. Heroine or smack is synthesized from crude opium (*afeem*) by making it to react with acetic anhydride. Other synthetic opioids that are frequently consumed include pentazocine, codeine, tramadol and dextropropoxyphene.

These substances act on the mu receptors present on the VTA and increase the concentration of dopamine in nucleus accumbens. These receptors are also present on the locus ceruleus which sends the noradrenergic projections to the whole brain, and this area is important for some of the withdrawal symptoms of opioids. Table 4.1.6 presents the clinical picture of opioid addiction.

NEUROBIOLOGY OF ADDICTION

Three processes—craving, tolerance and withdrawal symptoms—maintain addiction. In this section, we will discuss briefly the neurobiology related to all the three processes.

Addiction is the result of six different neuronal circuits that go dysfunctional. VTA sends dopaminergic projections to the nucleus accumbens and also to the prefrontal cortex. VTA increases the dopamine in these areas, but projections to the nucleus accumbens are more important for euphoria

Table 4.1.6. Clinical Picture of Opioid Addiction

Intoxication	Withdrawal	Use Disorder
Behavioural changes ranging from apathy to agitation, impairment of judgment along with pupillary constriction (however, during hypoxia, dilatation may be seen), drowsiness, coma, slurred speech and attention and memory impairment	Dysphoria, nausea, myalgia, pupillary dilation, watering from eye, sneezing with rhinorrhoea, diarrhoea, sweating, yawning, sleep disturbance Appears 1–3 days after the last intake of substance	All symptoms mentioned in 'use disorder' (see text);these patients are often constipated and take a long time to pass stool;they are involved in antisocial activities

(feeling of reward) associated with consumption of substances of abuse. However, with repeated administration, neuroadaptation occurs and less dopamine is released with further exposure (Fig. 4.1.1). To compensate it, they require higher doses of the substance.

Dorsal striatum is important for habit formation and glutaminergic signals from the cortex to the VTA, nucleus accumbens and substantia nigra enhance this habit formation. VTA also receives glutaminergic signals from nucleus accumbens (reward), insula (introception), hypothalamus (homoeostasis), amygdala (emotions) and orbitofrontal cortex (salience) which modulate its activity during exposure to paraphernalia (conditioned cues). This circuitry is important for drug craving; hence, these persons develop craving when they are exposed to the situations associated with drug use, eg, place from where they purchase the substance and persons with whom they consume it. In other words, craving heightens when the person is exposed to paraphernalia associated with substance use.

Prefrontal cortex is involved in decision-making and inhibitory behaviour. Addicted patients have lower availability of the dopamine receptors in this region, which reduces inhibitory control and increases drug seeking. This region is also important for the 'delay in gratification' and these subjects are not able to postpone gratification. Hence, they seek addictive substances to seek pleasure.

Circuitry involved in motivation (nucleus accumbens, anterior cingulate cortex, dorsolateral prefrontal cortex, dorsal striatum, orbitofrontal cortex and amygdala) is dysfunctional in these subjects and is governed by dopamine. It gets activated during the acts of drug seeking and this is why they remain engaged in behaviours involved in obtaining the drugs. In case of unavailability of the substance, they become uninterested in the surroundings.

Insula is an important region that provides internal sensory and autonomic inputs to the amygdala and nucleus accumbens and combines them with emotions. It has been found that people with damage to the insula can remain abstinent from drugs without craving for it, and thus they do not relapse after quitting the substance of abuse. Activity of this region may serve as a biomarker to predict the relapse.

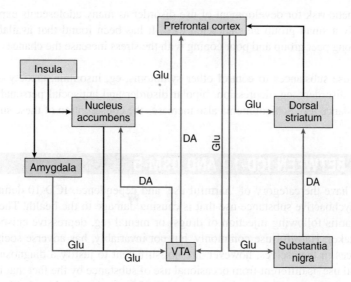

FIGURE 4.1.1

Neurocircuitry of addiction.

Habenula acts to reduce dopamine and thus, it has 'reward-antagonizing' action. Highly sensitive habenula reduces dopamine and thus increases the drug-seeking behaviour.

NEUROBIOLOGY OF TOLERANCE AND WITHDRAWAL

Contrary to the craving, tolerance and withdrawal are cellular processes and can be best understood depending upon the changes occurring at (1) subcellular level, ie, receptors and second messenger system, and (2) cellular level.

With continuous availability of the substance in the synaptic cleft, the receptors on the postsynaptic membrane reduce in number (internalize) or become less sensitive (desensitization) or uncouples with the second messenger system (eg, cAMP). Thus, the final output from the neuron or neuronal circuits is reduced and to achieve similar level of output a higher dose is required. This is the mechanism behind tolerance.

Continuous availability of the substance in the synaptic cleft, depending upon the action of substance, keeps the postsynaptic neuron in either excited or inhibited state. During withdrawal, the postsynaptic neurons start firing at a higher rate and thus, the effects that are opposite to the tolerance and intoxication are seen.

EPIDEMIOLOGY AND RISK FACTORS

The prevalence of use of these substances varies with geographical area, gender and age group. However, tobacco is perhaps the most commonly abused substance in India followed by alcohol or cannabis. Inhalant use is also increasing among the adolescents, however, its exact prevalence in India is not known.

There is a genetic risk for development of use disorder as many adolescents experiment with the substance but only a small group gets addicted to it. It has been found that availability of the substance, its use among peer group and poor coping with the stress increase the chances of indulging into substance use.

Many people use substances to control other symptoms, eg, insomnia, anxiety and chronic pain. Other psychiatric disorders, eg, depression, bipolar disorder and antisocial personality disorder, also predispose to substance use. Schizophrenia also increases the consumption of these substances.

DIFFERENCE BETWEEN ICD-10 AND DSM-5

DSM-5 does not have the category of 'harmful use' and dependence. ICD-10 defines 'harmful use' as a pattern of psychoactive substance use that is causing damage to the health. The damage may be physical (eg, hepatitis following injection of drugs) or mental (eg, depressive episodes secondary to heavy alcohol intake). Harmful use commonly, but not invariably, has adverse social consequences; social consequences in themselves, however, are not sufficient to justify a diagnosis of harmful use. However, 'harmful use' is different from occasional use of substance by the fact that it must persist for at least 1 month and must have recurred over a period of 12 months. On the other hand, 'dependence' is characterized by craving, lack of control, tolerance, withdrawal, preoccupation with the substance and consumption of substance despite knowing that it is harmful for the health. In DSM-5, both these conditions have been clubbed to 'use disorder'.

DIFFERENTIAL DIAGNOSIS

These disorders should be differentiated from nonpathological or nonproblematic use of substance, ie, sparing use of these substances. There may be an accidental exposure or continued use on the prescription, which should be differentiated.

DIAGNOSTIC FALLACIES

It is not uncommon for some people to use some of the medications for a long time after a single prescription, eg, sedatives—hypnotics and opiates. In these cases, other criteria for the 'use disorder' are often not met and they should not be diagnosed with substance use disorder.

Some medications, eg, hypnotics, stimulants may be prescribed for the medical reasons even for a fairly long duration. During weaning, some patients may experience withdrawal symptoms. However, they should not be given the diagnosis of substance withdrawal.

MANAGEMENT

It depends upon the state of addiction, ie, intoxication, use disorder and withdrawal. The type of substance in question also influences it.

Intoxication is primarily managed by supportive medical therapy. Inverse agonists are available for alcohol, benzodiazepines and opiates. They may be used during life-threatening intoxication, with the caution that they may precipitate severe withdrawal reactions. Naloxone, an opioid antagonist, may be used for opiate intoxication.

During withdrawal, pharmacological agonists should be used to control the pace of withdrawal, eg, benzodiazepines for alcohol (eg, oxazepam 10–60 mg/day; lorazepam 2–12 mg/day and opiates buprenorphine 2–8 mg/day; tramadol 50–200 mg/day) for the opioid withdrawal. Choice of a particular molecule depends upon the medical condition of the patient, half-life of the molecule and possible adverse effects.

Management of 'use disorder' is a two-step process. First step is detoxification where the patient is withdrawn from the substance and the withdrawal is managed. At the same time, medical problems are also investigated and addressed.

Once the detoxification is over, second phase starts where the patient is motivated for maintaining abstinence and, at the same time, comorbid psychiatric and medical disorders are addressed. Pharmacotherapy with long-acting substitutes, eg, methadone or buprenorphine, for opioid/opiates may be prescribed for the management of this phase.

Deterrents may also be used in selected cases after seeking informed consent, eg, disulfiram for alcohol. Another choice is to use anticraving drugs, eg, baclofen (found beneficial for all kinds of substances) or acamprosate for alcohol.

COURSE AND PROGNOSIS

Use of substances often starts with experimentation and biologically vulnerable people become addicted to it. 'Use disorder' often runs a chronic course with multiple lapses and relapses.

GAMBLING DISORDER

Gambling disorder is diagnosed when a person requires more money to achieve the same amount of excitement and becomes irritable when forbidden to do so. Other symptoms include gambling again even after losing a bet, a failure in stopping himself/herself from gambling and preoccupation with the thought of gambling. This habit causes significant distress in daily functioning. These people often steal money for the same, try to hide this habit and gamble when distressed. It starts often at a young age and at adulthood and progresses more rapidly among women as compared to men. Neurobiology is similar to that of addiction. It must be differentiated from gambling during a manic episode and antisocial personality disorder. Dopaminergic medications (those used during Parkinson disease and restless legs syndrome) may induce it. Naltrexone (50–100 mg/day) may be tried for the management of gambling disorder.

SUMMARY

- Addiction is a disease, not just a habit.
- Dysfunctional neurocircuitry is responsible for addiction.
- The disease has a typically chronic, relapsing course.
- Maintenance of sobriety is an achievable goal through treatment with judicious combination of pharmacological and psychosocial treatments.
- Behavioural addiction disorders are known and can be managed with medical help.

FURTHER READING

1. American Psychiatric Association. (2013). "Diagnostic and Statistical Manual of Mental Disorders." 5th edit, Author, Washington, DC.
2. Feduccia A. A., Chatterjee S., and Bartlett S. E. (2012). Neuronal Nicotinic Acetylcholine Receptors: Neuroplastic Changes Underlying Alcohol and Nicotine Addictions. *Frontiers in Molecular Neuroscience*, 5:83.
3. Jain R., and Balhara Y. P. (2008). Neurobiology of Cannabis Addiction. *Indian Journal of Physiology and Pharmacology*, 52:217–232.
4. Kosten T. R., and George T. P. (2002). The Neurobiology of Opioid Dependence: Implications for Treatment. *Science & Practice Perspectives*, 1:13–20.
5. Lubman D. I., Yücel M., and Lawrence A. J. (2008). Inhalant Abuse Among Adolescents: Neurobiological Considerations. *British Journal of Pharmacology*, 154:316–326.
6. Volkow N. D., and Baler R. D. (2014). Addiction Science: Uncovering Neurobiological Complexity. *Neuropharmacology*, 76(Pt B):235–249.
7. World Health Organization. (1992). "The ICD-10 Classification of Mental and Behavioural Disorders: Clinical Descriptions and Diagnostic Guidelines." Author, Geneva.

NEUROCOGNITIVE DISORDERS

5.1

Ravi Gupta

Neurocognitive disorders represent conditions where cognitive dysfunction is the primary pathology. Before we go into the details of each of these disorders, it is important that we understand what the term 'cognition' refers to! In simple words, cognition is our ability to gather all the information from the internal and external environment (*which requires a basal level of arousal, attention and concentration so that we can perceive*), process it in a meaningful manner (*which requires different types of memory systems—eg, working memory, retrieval of old information, ie, long-term memory; ability to compare the incoming information with that of the previous information, ie, abstraction and reasoning*) and reacting in an useful and contextually appropriate manner (*ie, planning and executive functioning*) (Fig. 5.1.1).

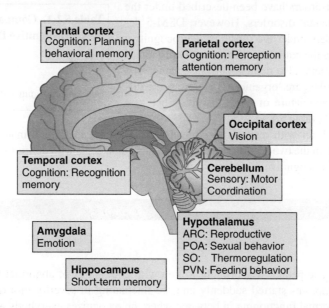

Frontal cortex
Cognition: Planning
behavioral memory

Parietal cortex
Cognition: Perception
attention memory

Occipital cortex
Vision

Temporal cortex
Cognition: Recognition
memory

Cerebellum
Sensory: Motor
Coordination

Amygdala
Emotion

Hypothalamus
ARC: Reproductive
POA: Sexual behavior
SO: Thermoregulation
PVN: Feeding behavior

Hippocampus
Short-term memory

FIGURE 5.1.1

Function of different brain areas. Functions are distributed across various areas of the brain and their coordinated functioning is required for even the simple tasks.

(Source: Menopause and Aging. Yen and Jaffe's Reproductive Endocrinology 2009. 10.1016/B978-1-4160-4907-4.00014-0.)

171

These functions are dependent upon different areas of the brain and thus, neurocognitive disorders can emerge in a variety of conditions that affect the functioning of the brain as we shall see in the subsequent paragraphs.

It must be noted that all psychiatric and neurological disorders emerge because of a functional and/or structural change in the brain; hence, they present with subtle cognitive dysfunction. For example, persons with schizophrenia and depression have slight cognitive problems. Similarly, patients having lacunar infarcts or early Parkinson disease also show cognitive dysfunction. However, as of now, the term neurocognitive disorders is limited to those disorders where the larger part of the clinical picture is cognitive dysfunction. Second, people with intellectual disability and neurodevelopmental disorders also present with focal or global dysfunction of cognitive process but they have *not* been included under the rubric of neurocognitive disorders. This term encompasses those disorders where there is a *decline in the level of previously achieved* cognitive functions. Last, the term 'cognition' has different meaning in medical literature and psychology. We have already explained its meaning with relation to medical literature; however, in psychology, its use is mostly limited to 'patterns of thinking'. Hence, you must note that 'cognitive behaviour therapy' has nothing to do with neurocognitive disorders.

So, by now, you are already equipped with the basic knowledge and we can proceed to acquire more knowledge regarding specific neurocognitive disorders.

NOSOLOGY

In ICD-10, these disorders have been described under the rubric of organic mental disorders. However, DSM-5 describes these disorders under the rubric of neurocognitive disorders, indicating the pathological process. Omission of term 'organic disorders' also depicts current concept that all psychiatric disorders are 'organic'. There are some differences in the nomenclature of these disorders between DSM-5 and ICD-10 (Table 5.1.1).

Table 5.1.1. Comparative Nosology of Neurocognitive Disorders

DSM-5	ICD-10
Delirium	Delirium
Major neurocognitive disorder	Dementia

Both disorders differ with respects to clinical picture, pathogenesis and management; hence, we have described them in the two sections separately. First section deals with delirium, whereas the second deals with major neurocognitive disorders.

DELIRIUM

VIGNETTE

A 40-year-old male patient was brought to you with complaints of abnormal behaviour since 2 days. The symptoms started suddenly and are fluctuating in severity in a day itself. There are periods of normal functioning in between where he recognizes everybody and behaves in a contextually appropriate manner. However, at other times, he starts yelling and talks to someone whom no one else can see. He is not able to recognize his family members and appears confused. He does not pay any attention when somebody talks to him and is making abnormal gestures. He has a history of chronic alcoholism and is abstinent for the past 6 months. He is a chronic smoker and was diagnosed with chronic obstructive pulmonary disease (COPD).

Family history was not contributory and he was not taking any medication during the past few days. Attendants of the patient confirmed that there was a clear deterioration in his awareness and attention during the past 5 days.

Clinical examination depicted laboured breathing, poor air entry in both sides of the lungs and multiple rhonchi on both sides of chest. Mental status examination revealed that he was confused. He was not oriented to time, place and person. Serial subtraction test (20-3 test) showed that although attention could be aroused, but it was ill sustained. 'Three words recall test' showed poor registration of information. Further examination of higher mental function was not possible. His psychomotor activity was increased, mood was irritable and what he was continuously muttering that was incomprehensible. He was making some gestures as if he was playing cards with his friends. He was poorly cooperative and detailed neurological examination was not possible. However, he did not have signs that could suggest cranial nerve or motor pathology. The diagnosis of 'acute delirium mixed level of activity, due to exacerbation of COPD' was made and further investigations were ordered.

CLINICAL PICTURE

The basic problem in delirium is the disturbance of attention and awareness of the surroundings, which evolved over hours to days. Attention cannot be aroused and even more difficult to sustain. Thus, these patients cannot hold information reaching to their brain. They appear confused and are disoriented to the surroundings and often make mistake in recognizing time, place or person. Resultantly, they may not provide an intended response to a given question. Sometimes, they keep on repeating one phrase in response to various questions (*perseveration*), because they are not able to shift their attention. In addition, one of the other faculties of neurocognitive functions is also involved. When memory is involved, the person is not able to register, retain or recall new information; when speech and language is involved, it is *incoherent* and sometimes *incomprehensible*; or person may experience *illusions or hallucinations*, where the perceptual ability is affected. The disturbance fluctuates during the course of the day. Symptoms may increase during night because of absence of external stimuli and some other yet to be explained reason (*sun downing*). However, patients who have delusions or perceptual disturbance may appear more agitated in the presence of external stimuli.

For better understanding and explanation of clinical picture, few specifiers have been added to the diagnosis of delirium.

Based on duration

When this clinical picture lasts for hours to days, it is termed '*acute*' and when such clinical picture continues beyond days, '*persistent*' specifier is added.

Based on psychomotor activity

At the same time, another specifier may be added depending upon the level of psychomotor activity. When it is increased from the baseline (ie, activity before the onset of delirium), it is called '*hyperactive delirium*' and when a reduction from the baseline is seen, it is termed '*hypoactive delirium*'. '*Mixed level of activity*' depicts that psychomotor activity is fluctuating during the course of illness.

Table 5.1.2 Causative Factors for the Development of Delirium

Metabolic and Endocrinal	Infections and Nutritional Deficiency	Disorders Affecting CNS	Substance Intoxication and Withdrawal
Hyponatraemia	Peritonitis	Head injury	Alcohol withdrawal
Hypernatraemia	Sepsis	Stroke	Hypnotic withdrawal
Hypokalemia	Meningitis	Tumours	Alcohol intoxication
Hyperkalemia	Encephalitis		Opioid intoxication
Hypoxia	Thiamine deficiency		Cannabis intoxication
Hypercarbia	Niacine deficiency		Cocaine intoxication
Acidosis or alkalosis			Nicotine intoxication
Hypoglycaemia			
Hepatic failure			
Renal failure			
Hypothyroidism			
Cushing syndrome			
Syndrome of inappropriate ADH secretion (SIADH)			

NEUROBIOLOGY

Delirium is a syndrome with multiple aetiologies (Table 5.1.2).

We have already seen that cognitive functions are dependent upon normal functioning of a number of areas of the brain. These areas are made up of neurons that communicate with each other through neurotransmitters. This exchange of information within a given area is responsible for a given cognitive faculty, eg, prefrontal cortex for immediate memory, orbitofrontal area for attention and planning and so on. However, different areas also communicate with each other so as to take a decision after examining the information from all aspects.

These cortical areas function normally when their tone is maintained by ascending reticular activating system (ARAS). ARAS arises from brainstem and is composed of various neurotransmitter nuclei—dopaminergic, noradrenergic, histaminergic, serotonergic and cholinergic to name a few. This basal tone maintains the arousal and makes us aware of surroundings. When the synthesis, storage, release, reuptake or catabolism of neurotransmitter is altered by any of the drugs (1, 2 and 4 in Fig. 5.1.2), neurotransmission gets altered, leading to delirium. Similar picture can emerge when drugs affect the postsynaptic functioning by altering the properties of postsynaptic neurons (3 in Fig. 5.1.2). This kind of picture can be seen in delirium caused by overdose of psychotropic drugs including substances of abuse—cocaine, stimulants, LSD, cannabis, alcohol and opium.

Our knowledge of neurophysiology tells us that, for normal functioning, like any other cell of the body, neurons also require energy, ie, ATPs. These ATPs are generated through metabolism of various substances and require many cofactors and trace elements. Moreover, these cells maintain a potential around the cell membrane for normal functioning and a reversible change in the membrane potential is observed during neurotransmission (5, 6 and 7 in Fig. 5.1.2). When the homoeostasis of the blood is altered, as we see during hyponatraemia, hypernatraemia, hypoglycaemia, hypoxaemia, renal failure and hepatic failure, functioning of the neurons gets altered, leading to desynchronized neurotransmission and emergence of delirium. Similar picture arises during deficiency of trace elements and vitamins (8 in

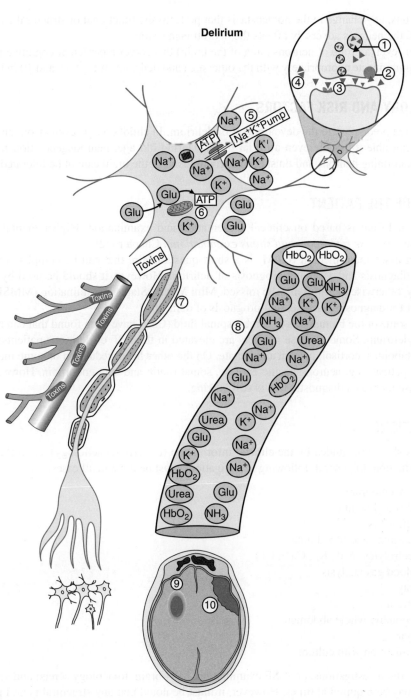

FIGURE 5.1.2

Neurobiology of delirium.

Fig. 5.1.2). Thus, any change in the homeostasis that perturbs the functional or structural environment in and around the neurons adversely affects the neurotransmission.

At a larger level, a group of neurons (area of the brain) that serves a particular cognitive function is not able to communicate appropriately with the other area and delirium emerges (9 and 10 in Fig. 5.1.2).

EPIDEMIOLOGY AND RISK FACTORS

Extremes of age predispose to the development of delirium. In childhood, it results from an immature brain that is not able to handle even a trivial insult. During old age, neurodegeneration reduces the number of functioning neurons and thus, even a trivial insult to the brain cannot be tolerated.

WORK-UP OF THE PATIENT

Diagnosis of delirium is based on clinical presentation and examination. Higher mental functions should be tested *(please refer to mental status examinationin* Chapter 1.2).

Confusion assessment method (CAM) is a short questionnaire that can be completed in 10 min and helps in diagnosis and assessing prognosis of delirium. However, it should be used by an expert clinician only, otherwise delirium may be missed. Mini Mental Status Eexamination (MMSE) is not a preferred tool for diagnosing or assessing prognosis of delirium.

Recently, some of the biomarkers in cerebrospinal fluid (CSF) have been found that can help in the diagnosis of delirium. Some of these markers are elevated in the CSF of delirious patients, eg, IL-8, serotonin metabolites, cortisol, protein and lactate. On the other hand, reduction of some markers was seen in these patients, eg, neuron-specific enolase, somatostatin and beta-endorphin. However, robust evidence to use them as a diagnostic tool is still lacking.

INVESTIGATIONS

Investigations should be guided by the clinical information (underlying aetiology), comorbidities and clinical examination. In general, following investigations must be done in all cases:

- Complete haemogram
- Peripheral blood picture
- Liver function tests
- Serum creatinine and blood urea
- Serum electrolytes (Na^+, K^+, Ca^{+2}, Cl^-)
- Arterial blood gas analysis
- Chest X-ray
- CT scan brain
- Ultrasonography: whole abdomen
- Blood sugar
- Urine examination with culture

Other specific investigations, eg, CSF examination, MRI brain, toxicology screen and serum vitamin assays, may be required at times. However, it must be noted that any structural neural pathology cannot predict the development of delirium.

DIFFERENTIAL DIAGNOSIS

Owing to the presence of hallucinations and delusions, it may be mistaken for schizophrenia and other psychotic disorders. However, altered consciousness that is seen in delirium, differentiates between the two.

It must be differentiated from malingering by atypical presentation of symptoms during malingering. Patients with factitious disorder may present with symptoms suggestive of delirium; however, in these cases, underlying aetiology for the delirium cannot be established.

Sometimes delirious patients may have intense anxiety and, on the other hand, patients suffering from acute stress disorder, which often follows a severe stress, show dissociative symptoms. Thus, acute stress disorder may be confused with delirium. However, history of exposure to a stressful event can help in differentiating between them.

Neurocognitive disorder (erstwhile dementia) usually evolves slowly, over month to years and attention and awareness is usually preserved until late in the course of illness. These aspects can help in differentiating it from delirium. However, when delirium is superimposed on neurocognitive disorder, it may be difficult to differentiate between the two.

Inattention is common in attention-deficit hyperactivity disorder (ADHD). Persons with ADHD have difficulty in sustaining their attention. It differs from delirium in the presence of adequate awareness of the environment and in the *absence* of *obvious* dysfunction in other cognitive abilities.

DIAGNOSTIC FALLACIES

Orientation to time, place and person means that patient should be able to differentiate between day and night and approximately guess what time of the day is it (when he is made to see outside an open window); he is able to recognize that he is in hospital (not necessarily the name of the hospital); and people around him by looking at their uniforms (a person wearing a white coat is a medical professional), respectively. Do you think a person who was brought unconscious to the hospital would be able to tell you the name of hospital or the doctor or a person in a closed room would be able to track the time of the day? Expecting such responses from a patient can add to the false-positive diagnosis of the delirium.

For bedside testing of memory, three dissimilar words may be used (eg, apple, sky and bus). If you are using three similar words, eg sky, airplane and cloud, person may make a mental picture and test loses reliability.

It is prudent to establish 'a decline in the level of attention and awareness' while diagnosing delirium. These patients always have a history of normal functioning before the onset of symptoms.

Hallucinations, delusions and change in psychomotor activity and mood are seen in patients with delirium. However, it should not be confused with psychosis, as attention and awareness of the surroundings are not impaired in psychosis.

A minimal level of arousal is important for the diagnosis of delirium; hence, it should not be diagnosed in comatose patients.

MANAGEMENT

The management may be divided into two parts—palliative management and treatment of underlying aetiology. Essentially, the aetiological factor should be treated and symptomatic management works as an adjuvant. The goal of palliative management is temporary reduction of symptom load and improving the safety of patient and caregivers.

Common guidelines for management are as follows:

Palliative management

1. Make sure that vitals remain in normal limits.
2. Maintain hydration and electrolytes within normal range.
3. Patients should be reoriented to the time of the day, place and environment gently and from time to time.
4. Sleep disturbance should be minimized. Hypnotics should be used judiciously as lorazepam has been found to worsen the course of delirium. Antipsychotic agents with sedating property (haloperidol and quetiapine) should be preferred.
5. Physical restrain may be provided to hyperactive patients. They may be kept in a secluded room to reduce environmental stimuli.
6. Antipsychotics in low dose may be given as and when required to hyperactive patients. They reduce the activity and induce sedation. Usually haloperidol is given (1.5–2.5 mg) in the gradually incremental doses. This is available in oral as well as parenteral formulation. Second generation antipsychotics, eg, risperidone (1–4 mg/day), quetiapine (25–50 mg/day) and olanzapine (2.5–5 mg/day), may also be used in small doses. In high doses, these drugs are more likely to produce adverse effects.
7. Anticholinesterase inhibitors (eg, donepezil 5–10 mg/day), NMDA blockers (eg, memantine 5–10 mg/day) and melatonin agonists (eg, remelteon 8–16 mg/day) have been found effective in management of delirium. They may be used if not contraindicated.

Application of initial four strategies (1–4) also helps in preventing delirium.

COURSE AND PROGNOSIS

It is an illness with abrupt onset as we have already discussed. A good recovery is expected in most of the cases, provided the underlying cause for the delirium is found. Mortality, in most of the cases, is ascribed to the improper management of the underlying cause. Patients having increased amount of acetylcholinesterase in CSF, usually have poor prognosis.

SUMMARY

- Preventive strategies should be used in high-risk group.
- Avoid centrally acting anticholinergics and other psychotropics. Psychotropics alter the neurotransmission at various levels and can worsen the situation.
- Minimize the number of drugs as far as possible. Multiple drugs may interact in an unpredictable manner to worsen the condition.
- Although palliative management is important, the improvement finally depends upon the recognition of aetiological factor and its correction.

NEUROCOGNITIVE DISORDER (NCD)

VIGNETTE

A 70-year-old woman was brought by her son because she gets lost in unfamiliar environments. He mentioned that for the past 6 years, he had noticed a gradual decline in her memory and daily functioning. Now she often forgets where she had kept her belongings and keeps searching them. When she is not able to find them, she becomes angry, frustrated and yells on the family members or sometimes curses herself. She eats food many times a day because she is not able to recall that she already had her food. For the same reason, she takes bath repeatedly. She keeps on repeating whatever she had already communicated. She has become disorganized and not able to take care of herself. She is not able to come to any decision when the family members discuss any problem with her. She often forgets names and is not able to cook. Whenever they organize a get-together at home, she is not able to plan all the necessary activities for the event. Her sleep is normal and she does not appear depressed. Now the family members have to assist her in daily chores. There is no history of any neurological illness or medical illness. The patient's mother also had similar problem at the age of 70 and it continued and worsened till she was alive. Clinical examination revealed normal vitals and absence of motor, sensory and cerebellar signs. She was oriented to time, place and person. Her attention was easy to arouse, but concentration was poor. Tests of memory (three word recall test) showed normal registration but poor recall after 3 min (short-term memory). She was not able to recall the details of the recently organized get-together in the family. She could not tell the way to the clinician's chamber from the hospital reception even though she came walking herself. She appeared distressed and refused to comply for further examination. Based on the history and examination, diagnosis of major neurocognitive disorder was made. A CT scan of the brain was ordered and it showed cerebral atrophy (Fig. 5.1.3).

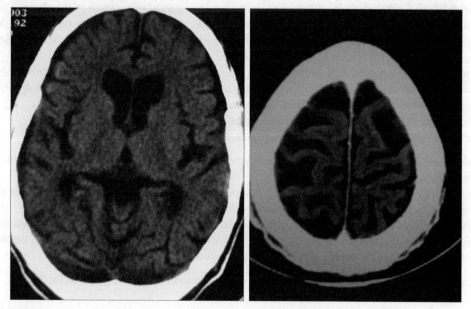

FIGURE 5.1.3

CT scan of the brain showing generalized prominent sulci due to cortical atrophy. (A) Lateral sulci are most affected and shrinkage of cerebellar folia is also seen. Ventricles are normal sized. (B) Sulcal widening showing cerebral atrophy.

(Source: *Himalayan Hospital, Dehradun*)

CLINICAL PICTURE

This is characterized by a decline in *at least one* of the cognitive functions, which is clinically significant. The decline from previous level of functioning should be a concern for individual himself, family members or the clinician. The clinical assessment or standardized cognitive testing must show a decline. These patients usually come with complaints that these days they tend to forget where they have kept their objects like keys and spectacles. They sometimes complain that they are not able to remember small grocery list of 5–6 items and frequently miss 1–2 items. They forget important events and dates that have happened in the past few days or months. People, who are in executive jobs, complain that they forget meetings, faces or names of people whom they have recently met (*memory*). Some of them adapt to failing memory by maintaining a diary or following a rigid schedule. To compensate the deficit, in the initial stage, they start keeping objects at a fixed place at home. They become disturbed and irritable upon asking them to deviate from their compensatory behaviours.

They are not able to plan their day or they may take a longer time than earlier to decide on complex issues or take the help of other people while dealing with complex issues (*planning and execution*). These patients are not able to do multitasking, which they were able to accomplish efficiently earlier (*complex attention*). Sometimes, these people have word-finding difficulty, which limits their performance (*language and speech*). Family members may complain of behaviours that are out of context or that the patient is now not able to understand the emotion of others (*social cognition*). When *visuospatial abilities* are involved, complaints are related with inability to navigate in a new environment or when the disease is severe, these people are lost even in familiar environment. There may be a decline in their ability to work with tools, cell phones or driving (*perceptual motor*)even in the absence of motor deficit. These features may arise because of an insult to the brain that may be related to a variety of factors, eg, age-related neurodegeneration, head injury, vascular insult or any other neurological disease like Parkinson disease and Huntington disease.

In the later stages, patient may become mute, apathetic, are not able to take care of themselves, incontinent and dependent upon the caregivers for day to day functioning. Sometimes they make obscene comments, make sexual advances (*social disinhibition*) when the frontal lobe functions become grossly deranged. Table 5.1.3 shows aetiological factors that can lead to neurocognitive disorders.

For better assessment of the illness, few specifiers have been added:

Mild NCD: When the decline in cognitive functions does not interfere with the person's ability to live independently on a day to day basis.
Major NCD: When the decline is so much that person is not able to live an independent life and frequently requires assistance to perform daily chores.
With behavioural symptoms: When symptoms like anxiety, depression, hallucinations or delusions, agitation, loss of motivation (apathy) or any other behavioural disturbance are associated with the NCD.
Without behavioural symptoms: Absence of behavioural symptoms.

Details regarding individual features of some of the common NCDs are given in Table 5.1.4.

NEUROBIOLOGY

Neurocognitive disorder is a syndrome with multiple aetiologies. As with delirium, it occurs owing to difficulty in neurotransmission within and across various brain areas that serve cognitive functions.

Table 5.1.3 Causes of Neurocognitive Disorder

Aetiology	Disorders	Type
Neurodegeneration	Alzheimer Disease Frontotemporal dementia Lewy body dementia Parkinson disease Huntington disease	Irreversible
Endocrinal	Hypothyroidism	Reversible
Nutritional	B1, B6 and B12 deficiency	Reversible
Vascular	Stroke Multiinfarct dementia	Partially reversible
Toxic	Alcohol dependence	Irreversible
Infections	HIV Encephalitis Prion disease Crutzfelds–Jacobs Disease	Irreversible
Injury	Head injury	May be reversible
Hydrocephalus	Normal pressure hydrocephalus	May be reversible

Many of these pathologies are reversible, eg, deficiency of vitamins (B1, B6 or B12), hypothyroidism and hydrocephalus. In some other cases, neurons suffer irreversible damage (infections, trauma, stroke and neurodegenerative illness) and once the problems setin, they are permanent or sometimes progressive (Table 5.1.4).

It is difficult to describe the pathophysiology of all of these disorders and here we will remain focused on one common problem—Alzheimer dementia. Some people are genetically predisposed to develop these illnesses and in them, the neurons start degenerating due to deposition of amyloid plaques inside them. These depositions are neurotoxic and they activate the pathways that lead to the damage of neurons through glutamate. Although almost all neurotransmitters are important for normal cognitive functioning, still the cholinergic nuclei of basal forebrain have been found most important for these functions. Damage to these cholinergic neurons has been reported in cases of Alzheimer disease (AD).

EPIDEMIOLOGY AND RISK FACTORS

In view of varying aetiologies, risk factors also vary. Here, we will focus on the risk factors associated with one of the commonest degenerative problem—AD. Increasing age and family history of neurocognitive disorders are two nonmodifiable risk factors. Risk increases after the age of 65 years and prevalence doubles every 5 years. After the age of 85 years, prevalence is around 50%. It tends to run in families and risk increases with increasing number of affected family members. It is related to transmission of genes that are responsible for development of symptoms across generations. Besides these two nonmodifiable factors, few risk factors are modifiable. Cardiovascular health is not only related to status of heart and stroke, but also, it increases the risk for developing AD. Thus, all the cardiovascular risk factors increase the risk for AD.

Table 5.1.4 Comparison of Different Neurocognitive Disorders Based on Aetiology

	Alzheimer Disease	Frontotemporal NCD	NCD with Lewy Bodies	NCD due to Parkinson Disease	Vascular NCD	NCD due to Traumatic Brain Injury (TBI)	Substance/Medication-Induced NCD	NCD due to HIV Infection	NCD due to Prion Disease	NCD due to Huntington Disease
Diagnosis	Memory and learning are first affected with or without executive functioning. Visuospatial ability and language are last to go. Social cognition is preserved until late in course.	*Behavioural variant* present with disinhibition, hyperorality, lack of sympathy and empathy, changed eating behaviours. Cognitive functioning less affected—poor planning, impaired judgment. Learning and memory relatively spared. *Language variant* presents with problems in word-finding, grammatical mistakes, comprehension of words and impaired speech production.	Decline in attention and executive functions appears first and fluctuates over time (*similar to delirium*). Hallucinations (often visual) and delusions appear. Memory and learning spared. Parkinson sets in approximately after a year. REM sleep behaviour disorder may be seen. Extreme sensitivity to neuroleptic drugs.	Decline in cognitive functioning after onset of Parkinson disease. Apathy, depression, anxiety or sleep disorders, like excessive daytime sleepiness and REM sleep behaviour disorder, may accompany.	Decline in complex attention and executive functioning appearing after a stroke	Cognitive decline after a TBI. TBI is diagnosed when history of head injury is accompanied by at least one of the following: loss of consciousness; posttraumatic amnesia; posttraumatic delirium; or neurological signs/neuroimaging demonstrating injury.	NCD is seen in patients abusing substance/medication for a sufficient time. Substance intoxication and withdrawal must be ruled out. Often improve after abstinence. Seen with alcohol, sedative hypnotics and inhalants.	Presentation varies depending upon the area of the brain involved. In general, presents with difficulty in learning, attention, executive functioning and slowing of processing.	Cognitive decline is associate with movement problems, eg, ataxia, myoclonus, dystonia, chorea. Seizures may be seen and patients may complain of startle reflex. Associated with Crutzfelds-Jacobs disease (CJD) and Kuru.	Memory is relatively preserved with loss of planning, organization and speed of processing the information. Associated with clinical picture of Huntington disease—bradykinesia or chorea (see Video 2).

Age of onset	Usually after 60 years	Before 65 years	Elderly	Elderly	Can appear at any age, but increases after 65 years.	Any age	Any age	Any age	Any age during adulthood	Approximately 40 years. But dependent upon the length of CAG repeats.
Course	Gradual onset and progressive course	Gradual onset and progressive course	Gradual onset and progressive	Gradual onset, progressive	Sudden onset. Course varies and dependent upon vascular insults.	Sudden onset. Variable course.	Variable. Cognitive deficits may improve after abstinence or may remain stable.	Variable, may fluctuate, resolve completely, improve to some extent or gradually progress.	Progressive	Gradually progressive
Pathology	Taupathy. Altered processing of amyloid precursor protein and formation of neuritic plaques.	Picks bodies (not in all)	Alpha-synucleopathy. Lewy bodies appear first in cortical areas and then in basal ganglia.	Alpha synucleopathy	Cerebrovascular pathology is evident.	Traumatic brain injury evident.	Varied, depending upon the substance.	Neuronal degeneration	Neuronal damage	CAG trinucleotide repeats. Basal ganglia mainly affected
Diagnostic markers	Mutation of APP, PSEN1 and PSEN2 gene in early onset familial cases.	Mutations of MAPT, GRN, TDP-43, VCP. FUS genes in familial cases.	None	None	None	None	None	Evidence of HIV-1 infection.	14-3-3 protein and Tau protein in CSF (For CJD). EEG shows periodic sharp waves.	CAG trinucleotide repeats.

Continued

Table 5.1.4 Comparison of Different Neurocognitive Disorders Based on Aetiology—Cont'd

	Alzheimer Disease	Frontotemporal NCD	NCD with Lewy Bodies	NCD due to Parkinson Disease	Vascular NCD	NCD due to Traumatic Brain Injury (TBI)	Substance/Medication-Induced NCD	NCD due to HIV Infection	NCD due to Prion Disease	NCD due to Huntington Disease
Neuroimaging	Cortical and hippocampal atrophy on CT/MRI. Functional imaging show reduced activity in temporoparietal cortices.	Frontotemporal atrophy on CT/MRI. Functional imaging shows hypometabolism in these areas.	Relatively preserved medial temporal lobe on CT/MRI. Low dopamine transporter uptake in striatum on PET/SPECT. Polysomnography for REM sleep behaviour disorder.	Similar to the NCD due to Lewy Bodies.	CT/MRI shows evidence of stroke.	CT/MRI suggests TBI.	MRI shows cortical atrophy with or without white matter abnormalities.	MRI shows atrophy.	MRI brain with diffusion weighed imaging shows multifocal grey matter hyperintensities.	MRI brain shows loss of volume in caudate and putamen.

WORK-UP OF THE PATIENT

Diagnosis is dependent upon the clinical information and patient's examination. Patient's complete neurological examination should be done as it may provide clues to the underlying aetiology. Higher mental functions should be tested (*please refer to history taking and examination in* Chapter 1.2). Some brief screening tools are available with different psychometric properties. Depending upon the need, availability and ease of use one of the following tools may be chosen:

- Mini mental status examination
- Modified mini mental status examination
- General practitioner assessment of cognition
- Mini cognitive assessment instrument
- Clock drawing test

Extended cognitive test batteries are sometimes required for the diagnosis. They also provide an objective assessment of level of functioning.

However, in some cases, laboratory investigations are required and the choice of investigation is guided by the clinical picture. It is prudent to differentiate between reversible and irreversible pathologies through appropriate method. In general, following investigations should be done in all the following cases:

- Thyroid profile
- Serum B12
- MRI scan of the brain
- EEG

Biomarkers can help in substantiating diagnosis of degenerative pathologies; however, their description is out of scope of this book. However, it must be remembered that the final diagnosis is histopathological and can be done on autopsy only.

DIFFERENTIAL DIAGNOSIS

Delirium should be differentiated by acute onset of illness, fluctuating course, loss of awareness to the surrounding and primary difficulty being attention. Although these features may be present in NCD, but they are seen only in later stages. When these features are present, possibility of delirium superimposed on NCD must be ruled out.

Intellectual disability and neurodevelopmental disorders can be distinguished by their presence since birth and retarded development cognitive functions. On the other hand, NCD shows a decline in the level of previously normal cognitive functions.

Mild NCD may sometimes be difficult to differentiate from normal cognition. In such cases, patient should be followed up sequentially to confirm the diagnosis.

Major depressive disorder may be difficult to differentiate from mild NCD. Different NCDs are associated with a specific decline in some areas of cognitive functions (eg, memory and execution in AD), whereas nonspecific areas are involved in depression.

DIAGNOSTIC FALLACIES

Symptoms and thus diagnosis may be missed, at least in the initial stage, in the patients who do not require intense cognitive functioning for their routine works, eg, drivers and labour. On the other hand, it may sometimes be over-diagnosed in high functioning individuals, eg, executives who keep a close watch on a minor change in their cognitive functioning.

Objective tests are also not immune from false-positive or false-negative diagnosis. High-functioning individuals may do well on cognitive tests (false-negative) or a 'low-functioning' person may not be able to perform even in the presence of normal functioning (false-positive).

Since, caregiver's concern is also important for the diagnosis, the diagnosis may be missed when family members are not able to perceive a change in cognitive functioning or when the patient himself has poor insight. Similarly, people who are excessively concerned with their health, keep a track of minor changes and may get a false diagnosis.

The diagnosis may be missed in persons when activities are limited because of any other reason, eg, an illness.

MANAGEMENT

The goal of treatment is the recovery of functional, behavioural and cognitive functions. Since, it is a condition with varied aetiologies, the treatment is directed towards the individual aetiology that has been found responsible for NCD. However, in general, it consists of behavioural and environmental manipulations along with pharmacotherapy. Both the therapies are important and best are instituted together. We will describe each of these therapies one by one.

A number of environmental and behavioural manipulations can help the patient to cope up with the decline in cognitive functioning. Some of these are listed below:

1. These patients should be encouraged to use compensatory strategies, eg, keeping a diary to remember the list of works, using the calculator for calculations and so on.
2. When these subjects have visuospatial disabilities, they may be provided with navigation tools so that they can find their ways.
3. It is better to keep them in a structured and familiar environment. Frequent changes in the location of their belongings in home or their own place of stay make them disoriented.
4. When the patient finds it difficult to navigate even at home, markers and direction signs may be stuck even in house so that they are able to find their ways.
5. They may be encouraged to refrain from toxins, eg, tobacco or alcohol.

PHARMACOTHERAPY

Anticholinesterase inhibitors increase the availability of acetylcholine in synapse and thus improve the symptoms. A variety of molecules (donapezil and rivastigmine) are available that can be used (Table 5.1.5).

Memantine blocks the ionotropic glutamate receptors and thus help in preventing injury and damage of neurons. This may be given with or without achicholinesterase inhibitors.

Psychotropics (antidepressants, antipsychotics and anxiolytics) may be used for management of behavioural symptoms.

COURSE AND PROGNOSIS

The course is variable and depends upon the underlying aetiology. Reversible dementias reverse as soon as the aetiology is addressed. Irreversible dementias usually have a progressive course since they are associated with neuronal damage.

Table 5.1.5 Drugs used for the Treatment of Neurocognitive Disorders

Class of Drug	Name of the Drug	Dose	Major Adverse Effects
Anticholinesterase inhibitors	Donapezil	5–10 mg/day	Headache, nausea, vomiting, agitation, cardiac arrhythmia, acidity and hepatitis
	Galantamine	8–12 mg/day	Nausea, vomiting, diarrhoea, agitation and hallucinations
	Rivastigmine	Upto 12 mg/day	Nausea, vomiting, bradycardia, syncope and hallucinations
NMDA receptor antagonist	Memantine	5–20 mg/day	Hypotension and dyspnoea

SUMMARY

- Neurocognitive disorders affect higher mental functioning.
- They are usually seen in elderly, but may present at an early age.
- Their diagnosis banks upon the decline in cognitive functioning which may be stable, progressive or reversible.

FURTHER READING

1. American Psychiatric Association. (2013). "Diagnostic and Statistical Manual of Mental Disorders." 5th edit, Author, Washington, DC.
2. Bishara D., Sauer J., and Taylor D. (2015). The Pharmacological Management of Alzheimer's Disease. *Progress Neurology and Psychiatry*, 19:9–16.
3. World Health Organization. (1992). "The ICD-10 Classification of Mental and Behavioral Disorders: Clinical Descriptions and Diagnostic Guidelines." Author, Geneva.

EPILEPSY AND SEIZURE DISORDERS

5.2

Ravi Gupta

'Seizure' refers to an abnormal, hypersynchronous electrical discharge from the brain, whereas 'convulsion' denotes abnormal, episodic, stereotyped movements, which may be on clonic or tonic type. Another term,'epilepsy' confers a clinical disorder where the person has repeated episodes of convulsions and seizures.

Epilepsy and convulsions are an important part of psychiatry practice. You may see a number of conditions that need to be differentiated from epilepsy, eg, convulsions occurring during the course of functional neurological symptoms disorders, which is also known as pseudo-seizures or nonepileptic seizures. However, if you closely look at the definition of 'seizure', you will find that terms like 'pseudo-seizures' and 'nonepileptic seizures' are misnomers as what we clinically see is a convulsion with normal electroencephalogram (EEG without seizures) and hence, better term would be nonepileptic convulsions. In addition, patients with epilepsy have a range of psychiatric symptoms ranging from psychosis and anxiety to mood disturbances. Similarly, nocturnal epilepsy should be differentiated from parasomnias (kindly refer to Chapter 6.1 on sleep disorders).

In this chapter, we will discuss the classification of seizures, their differential diagnosis and psychiatric disorders that may accompany epilepsy.

VIGNETTE

A 17-year-old girl was brought to the emergency department with recurrent episodes of loss of consciousness. Loss of consciousness in each episode lasted for approximately 2 h. They have been occurring in the school since past 2 months with a frequency of four to five episodes per week. During the episode, the girl used to fall down, although she was never injured. Then she developed some abnormal movements in the form of thrashing of limbs and clenching of fists and jaws. This used to last for around 1 h. At that time, the girl was not able to communicate with anyone. There was no history to suggest involuntary voiding or defecation, amnesia, tongue bite, progressive tonic-clonic movements during the episode. When interviewed, she told that she was aware of what was happening in the surroundings but was unable to communicate to the people. General physical and neurological examination did not add anything. Mental status examination disclosed distressed mood. Based on the history and examination, diagnosis of functional neurological symptoms disorder was made.

CLINICAL PICTURE

Epilepsy is generally classified into two major subtypes—generalized and partial. Generalized epilepsy refers to seizures occurring in the whole of brain and thus clinically it may manifest as generalized symptoms with loss of consciousness. On the other hand, in partial epilepsy, there is a focal onset of seizures, thus symptoms are localized. This type of epilepsy may be associated with loss of consciousness (complex partial seizures) or without it (simple partial seizures). When we talk about the loss of consciousness during a seizure, it actually means *reduced awareness to the surroundings*. Thus, a person with complex partial seizure may not exhibit commonly believed symptoms of unconsciousness (fall with eyes closed as we see in syncope), rather he remains unaware of the surroundings for the ictal period. As we have already discussed in Chapters 1.2 and 5.1, different brain areas regulate higher mental functions in a coordinated manner to keep us aware of the surroundings. Involvement of these areas during the epilepsy leads to unconsciousness.

Classification of epilepsy has been outlined in Table 5.2.1.

Detailed account of the semiology of the seizures is out of the scope of this book. For this, you may refer to a textbook of medicine or neurology. In this chapter, we will focus on the psychiatric aspects of epilepsy.

Table 5.2.1 Classification of Epilepsy (International League Against Epilepsy)	
1. Generalized	
1.1 Convulsive	Tonic–clonic–tonic Tonic-clonic
1.2 Absence seizures	Typical Myoclonic absence Eyelid myoclonia Atypical
1.3 Tonic	
1.4 Atonic	
1.5 Myoclonic	Myoclonic Negative myoclonic Myoclonic tonic Myoclonic atonic
2. Focal/partial	
2.1 By features	Motor Dyscognitive Aura Autonomic
2.2 Hemisphere localization	
2.3 Lobar localization	Frontal Temporal Parietal Occipital
Source: *https://www.epilepsydiagnosis.org/index.html (last accessed 31 July 2015).*	

EPILEPSY AND PSYCHIATRIC DISORDERS

Epileptic patients are at risk for development of psychiatric disorders, particularly psychosis and mood disorders. Psychiatric manifestations in epilepsy could be preictal, ictal, postictal and, lastly, interictal.

Prodrome consists of symptoms that are seen before the onset of a seizure. These manifestations are often nonspecific and include headache, loss of concentration, anxiety and dysphoria. Though they have been reported in cases of generalized epilepsy, yet they are more common among patients with focal epilepsy.

Aura and automatism depict the ictal psychiatric manifestation of epilepsy. Aura appears because of focal change in the neuronal activity. Thus, its symptoms vary with the location of the lesion. This can also help in localization of the epileptic foci. Aura may present as hallucinations (when it involves cortical areas that represent special senses), jerking or myoclonus (when involves motor cortex) or sense of derealization or depersonalization (when involves temporal lobe).

Automatism refers to the involuntary and repetitive motor activity that is seen in epilepsy patients. When asked afterwards, patients are not able to recall these activities. These activities include lip smacking, pursing of lips, licking, chewing, grimacing, laughing, crying and making gestures.

Postictal manifestations include postictal delirium that lasts for a variable period ranging from few minutes to few hours. For the symptoms of delirium, please refer to Chapter 5.1. Another psychiatric manifestation is postictal psychosis (*vide infra*).

Interictal manifestations of seizures include a variety of psychiatric syndrome, eg, anxiety, depression and psychosis. In DSM-5 and ICD-10, these disorders are termed as 'disorder secondary to the medical disorders'.

ANXIETY

Two of the anxiety disorders, ie, generalized anxiety disorder and phobia, are more common among patients with epilepsy. Many patients remain anxious of having a seizure at inappropriate places and hence they avoid going alone. These beliefs are irrational in these patients and hence, they qualify for the diagnosis of agoraphobia.

DEPRESSION AND BIPOLAR DISORDER

Depression is seen with higher frequency in epileptic patients as compared to the general population during the interictal period. It usually manifest as dysphoria rather than depressed mood. This has led to the origin of terms like interictal dysphoric disorder. Somatic symptoms like lack of energy and generalized pain are also common. Many of these patients have short symptom-free intervals and some may experience episodes of manic features as well. Besides, the neurobiological disturbances owing to epilepsy, antiepileptic drugs may also manipulate neurotransmission and cause depression. In particular, bariturates, vigabatrin and topiramate are known to be associated with depression in these patients.

PSYCHOSIS

Psychosis in epilepsy patients may take one of the two courses. It may be postictal psychosis where psychotic symptoms emerge in the background of increased seizure activity (recent increase in frequency of seizures). This activity is followed by a symptom-free period of few hours to days, following which psychotic symptoms appear. Clinically, it is manifested by presence of delusions (paranoid or grandiose), change in the mood and hallucinations. It lasts from few hours to few days. Many of these patients may be mistaken for the psychosis unless they develop a seizure. They often do not respond to antipsychotics. Hence, patients who do not respond to adequate dose of antipsychotic for adequate duration should be screened for epilepsy.

During the interictal period, patients with epilepsy may present with symptoms described in schizophrenia. When the symptoms are episodic, treatment consists of antiepileptic drugs only; however, when the symptoms are chronic, antipsychotics should be added to the antiepileptic drugs.

DIFFERENTIAL DIAGNOSIS OF SEIZURES

Seizures must be differentiated from a variety of conditions that include syncope, parasomnias, psychiatric disorders, paroxysmal movement disorders and migraine-associated features. Table 5.2.2 provides the details of epilepsy imitators. They should be differentiated from these disorders by history, clinical examination and appropriate investigations, eg, awake EEG or long-term video EEG or overnight video-synchronized EEG and neuroradiological investigations, like CT scan or MRI scan of the brain with epilepsy protocol.

One important condition that must be differentiated from seizures is nonepileptic convulsions. Nonepileptic convulsions are seen during functional neurological symptom disorder and they differ from true seizures in a variety of manners. These are listed in Table 5.2.3.

MANAGEMENT

In this section, we will focus on the treatment of psychiatric symptoms. Preictal and ictal manifestations may be improved by optimizing the control of seizure activity. Postictal delirium and postictal psychosis are self-limiting conditions and do not require any treatment. However, when the symptoms become severe, benzodiazepine (lorazepam 2–6 mg parenteral) may be prescribed.

Table 5.2.2 Imitators of Seizures

Psychiatric Condition	Seizure Mimics
Daydreaming and inattention	Absence seizures
Panic attacks	Autonomic seizures
Hallucinations, dissociative disorders	Temporal lobe seizures, aura
Sleep-related rhythmic movement disorders	Nocturnal epilepsy
Other parasomnias	Complex partial seizures
Cataplexy	Atonic seizures
Migraine with visual aura	Occipital epilepsy
Tics and other paroxysmal movement disorders	Focal seizures

Table 5.2.3 Differentiation Between Nonepileptic Convulsion and True Seizure

	Nonepileptic Convulsion	True Seizure
Settings	Occurs when people are around, usually after a stressful event, rarely during sleep unless the patient wakes up during sleep.	Occurs irrespective of these symptoms.
Premonitory symptoms	Usually absent.	May be seen, usually mood disturbances or cognitive may start 1–2 days before the attack.
Aura	Absent.	May be reported in cases of focal seizures or focal with secondary generalization. Symptomatology vary depending upon the origin of seizures.
Attack	Usually long, movements are not stereo-types, they are usually coarse, instead of true tonus, clenching of fists and jaw is seen. Pelvic thrusting is seen instead of true clonic movements. Seldom the patient gets injured, tongue bite almost never seen, involuntary defecation or voiding rarely seen.	Usually short, lasts for few minutes, regains consciousness after 10–20 min. Movements progress from one part of the body to other, true tonic or clonic and vary depending upon the type of epilepsy. Patients usually falls resulting in injury, tongue bite, involuntary micturition or defecation.
Postictal period	Patient often remains unconscious for hours after the attack.	Short. Patient appears delirious after the attack that clears within few hours. May complain of generalized fatigue or headache.
Examination	Intraictal EEG normal; postictal prolactin normal; deep tendon reflexes normal or exaggerated; planter reflex is flexor.	Intraictal EEG shows epileptic discharges; prolactin elevated; planter often extensor.

Anxiety disorders can be managed by judicious use of long-acting benzodiazepines (eg, clonazepam 0.5–1 mg/day) along with cognitive behaviour therapy.

When you encounter patients with interictal depression, consider a recent change in the antiepileptic drugs that may be responsible for depression (bariturates, vigabatrin and topiramate). Valproate and carbamazepine have beneficial effects in depression and they may be started in these patients. If the patients show severe symptoms, antidepressants may be started. The selective serotonin reuptake inhibitors (escitalopram 5–10 mg/day or sertraline 25–100 mg/day) remain the drug of choice owing to their adverse-effect profile. In many cases, treatment of depression improves seizure control.

Interictal psychosis can be treated with drugs that have low-seizure potential, eg, haloperidol and risperidone, in optimal doses.

SUMMARY

- Epilepsy patients are at higher risk for psychiatric disorders.
- Behavioural symptoms seen during premonitory, preictal, ictal and postictal phases may mimic psychiatric disorders.
- Psychiatric disorders may mimic epilepsy.
- Management of both behavioural symptoms as well as epilepsy is important for improving the quality of life of the patient.

FURTHER READING

1. http://www.ilae.org/Visitors/Centre/Definition-2014-Perspective.cfm(accessed on 19July2015).
2. http://onlinelibrary.wiley.com/doi/10.1111/j.1528-1167.2011.03101.x/full(accessed on 19July2015).
3. https://www.epilepsydiagnosis.org/epilepsy-imitators.html#tantrums(accessed on 19July2015).
4. Mellers J. D. C. Epilepsy. In "Lishman's Organic Psychiatry: A Textbook of Neuropsychiatry"(A. S. David, S. Fleminger, M. D. Kopelman, S. Lovestone, J. D. C.Mellers, Eds.). 4th Edit. pp. 309–396. Wiley-Blackwell, Chichester, West Sussex, England.

ANTI-NMDA RECEPTOR ENCEPHALITIS

5.3

Ravi Gupta

Anti-NMDA receptor encephalitis is a disorder that belongs to the group of autoimmune diseases where antibodies are formed against neuronal receptors. Till date, antibodies have been discovered against various neuronal receptors, eg, N-methyl-D-aspartate receptor (NMDAR), alpha-amino-3-hydroxy-5-methylisoxazole-4-proprionic acid receptors (AMPAR), GABA$_B$ receptors, glycine receptors and potassium channel-associated complex. This disorder was discovered in 2005. However, amongst all these neuronal receptors, anti-NMDAR encephalitis is most common, hence we will discuss it in this chapter.

VIGNETTE

The family members of a 23-year-old woman with complaints of altered behaviour brought her after the remission of fever. The woman appeared anxious and was fearful. Her family members reported that she had complained of hearing some voices that nobody else could hear. She had also become suspicious and was not eating anything at home because she feared that they were trying to poison her. Symptoms were seen for the past 7 days and were increasing in severity. Her sleep–wake cycle was also altered and, at times, she appeared confused. General physical and neurological examination was within normal limits. Mental status examination revealed dysphoric mood, auditory hallucinations and delusion of persecution. Based on the history and examination, working diagnosis of anti-NMDA receptor encephalitis was made.

CLINICAL PICTURE

It is most commonly seen in young females; however, no age group and gender is immune. In the prodromal phase, patients often present with symptoms of influenza; hence, they seek consultation of a general physician or a paediatrician. However, after 15 days of influenza, these patients may develop psychotic symptoms, ie, delusions and hallucinations, anxiety, apathy, depression and change in neurocognitive functioning. Some patients may have abnormal involuntary movements or seizures. Next, patients become catatonic with inappropriate smiling and then they may enter a phase of hyperkinesia that is characterized by dyskinesia and appearance of extrapyramidal features. Contrary to psychosis, these patients have fluctuating levels of consciousness that clinically appears as delirium. Time course from the onset to appearance of various symptoms may vary.

NEUROBIOLOGY

Anti-NMDAR encephalitis interferes with the glutaminergic communication owing to internalization of its receptor, leading to the production of various psychiatric symptoms that may be confused with psychosis and schizophrenia.

This disorder is often associated with ovarian tumours and teratomas. However, in many cases, it is not found because it may be below the level of detection. In those cases, where you find an evidence of the tumour, removal of tumour may terminate the symptoms. It is also possible that infectious agents interact with the tumour cells to produce an antibody against NMDAR.

DIAGNOSIS

Diagnosis is difficult, as MRI of the brain do not show any abnormality in half of the cases. In other cases hyperintensity on T2 and FLAIR imaging may be seen. Laboratory diagnosis involves detection of antibodies against NMDAR through cell-based assays. Patient's serum may be used to detect antibody and if it turns out to be negative, cerebrospinal fluid may be taken as the source of NMDAR antibodies.

MANAGEMENT

Treatment includes acyclovir unless the herpes simplex encephalitis is excluded. Seizures may be controlled using anticonvulsants. After confirming the diagnosis, this should be treated on the lines of autoimmune disorders with use of corticosteroids, plasma exchange and use of monoclonal antibodies. Psychiatric symptoms must be managed depending upon the symptomatology, as described in various chapters.

COURSE AND PROGNOSIS

Many of the patients improve with supportive therapy; however, in some cases, disease may take a long course with residual neurocognitive impairment and frontal lobe syndrome.

SUMMARY

- NMDA receptor encephalitis mimics psychotic disorders.
- A high index of suspicion is required to diagnose this illness.
- Therapy targeted at resolution of autoimmune pathology is effective in its management.

FURTHER READING

1. Peery H. E., Day G. S., Dunn S., Fritzler M. J., Prüss H., De Souza C., Doja A., Mossman K., Resch L., Xia C., Sakic B., Belbeck L., and Foster W. G. (2012). Anti-NMDA Receptor Encephalitis. The Disorder, the Diagnosis and the Immunobiology. *Autoimmunity Reviews*.doi:10.1016/j.autrev.2012.03.001

STROKE

Ravi Gupta

Stroke leads to a variety of psychiatric symptoms that range from mood disorders to cognitive impairment. Thus, as a neuropsychiatrist you may be called to manage these issues. All of us know following two facts— first, stroke leads to damage in the affected areas of the brain and second, that all psychiatric disorders are neurobiological. Thus, neuronal damage consequent to stroke may affect neurotransmission across various pathways and communication across various areas of the brain, leading to the emergence of psychiatric symptoms. In this chapter, we will discuss common psychiatric conditions seen after a stroke.

VIGNETTE

A 72-year-old man presented with history of loss of interest in daily activities, sad mood, loss of appetite and decreased sleep for 1 month. He reported that symptoms developed after he had suffered a stroke 3 months back. He did not have any other medical illness or a past history of psychiatric disorders. However, his mother had suffered multiple episodes of depression. General physical examination was not contributory to the diagnosis. Neurological examination revealed hemiparesis on the left side. Mental status examination depicted decreased psychomotor activity, sad mood and depressed thoughts. CT scan of the brain depicted stroke in the right occipital lobe. Based on the history and examination, diagnosis of post-stroke depression was made (Fig. 5.4.1).

CLINICAL PICTURE

In this section, we will discuss regarding the common disorders that may appear in association with stroke and their management.

CATASTROPHIC REACTION

It appears acutely after the stroke in around one-fifth of the patients. These patients have a family history of psychiatric disorders. Catastrophic reaction may be associated with major depressive disorder. Contrary to common belief, it does not have any relationship with aphasia. These patients present with intense anxiety and aggression. Some of them develop depressive symptoms.

PATHOLOGICAL EMOTIONS

Some of the patients may present with episodes of crying or laughter that may be inappropriate to the context. These emotions may be provoked by trivial stimulus, but these patients deny having similar feelings. This is also termed as pseudo-bulbar affect. Tricyclics have been found to be effective in management of these symptoms.

POST-STROKE DEPRESSION

Nearly half of the stroke patients develop depression that may last up to 1 year. The symptoms of depression do not differ from that of major depressive disorder seen without stroke (please refer to depressive disorders in Chapter 3.1). These patients often have stroke in the left anterior regions. Depression in stroke patients is often associated with physical disability. However, disability is not causal to depression; rather, literature suggests that post-stroke depression increases the physical disability, which can be improved by early improvement for the depression. Selective serotonin reuptake inhibitors may be used for the management of post-stroke depression.

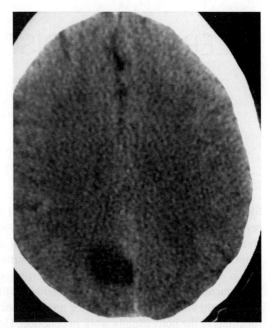

FIGURE 5.4.1

CT scan showing infarct in the right occipital lobe.
(Source: Himalayan Hospital, Dehradun)

POST-STROKE MANIA

Symptoms of mania in these patients are similar to those of without stroke (please refer to bipolar disorders in Chapter 3.1). It is more common with right anterior lesions. Family history of mood disorders may be a risk factor for this condition. Mood stabilizers have been found effective in the treatment of post-stroke mania.

POST-STROKE NEUROCOGNITIVE DISORDER

Stroke can produce cognitive impairment by damaging the neurons (please refer to Chapter 5.1 on neurocognitive disorders). Symptoms are similar to neurocognitive disorder although they may vary depending upon the location of the lesion. However, cognitive symptoms may be patchy depending upon the area involved; in cases with recurrent strokes, symptoms may appear in a progressive fashion along with other neurological symptoms.

SUMMARY

- Stroke, by damaging various brain areas, can produce psychiatric symptoms.
- Psychiatric symptoms may influence recovery from stroke.

SLEEP AND ITS DISORDERS

6.1

Ravi Gupta

Sleep can be understood as a state of perceptual disengagement to and from the environment that is reversible in response to any internal or external stimulus. As you already know that wakefulness and sleep are the two states of consciousness, which are governed by the neurotransmitter systems of the brain, primarily the monoaminergic system. Furthermore, sleep itself consists of four different stages, which evolve because of the complex interplay of these neurotransmitter systems, as we shall see subsequently. In addition, it must be remembered that physiological functions alter during sleep so as to maintain the sleep and match with the metabolic needs of the body. Thus, sleep and other physiological functions of the body usually work in cohesion. However, sometimes sleep becomes disordered due to changes in the brain and this can have a negative influence on the body, eg, diabetes and cardiovascular disorders are more common among insomnia as compared to normal sleepers. On the other hand, alteration in the physiological functions may also alter the sleep quality or quantity, eg, congestive heart failure induces Cheyenne–Stokes breathing and this leads to poor sleep quality. In this chapter, we will discuss about the physiology of sleep and its common disorders.

PHYSIOLOGY OF SLEEP

As we have already discussed, sleep is an active process. It is governed by two independent factors—homoeostatic factors and circadian factors (Fig. 6.1.1). Homoeostatic factors increase 'sleep pressure', which means, the longer we are awake, the higher the sleep pressure. Thus, it is lowest in the morning and further reduces after a nap. During sleep deprivation, it is this pressure that keeps on accumulating and thus we tend to fall asleep even involuntarily. This deprivation can be complete (after no sleep at all) or partial (eg, cutting few hours of sleep from usual sleep duration). On the other hand, circadian factors regulate the sleep–wake cycle with reference to the environmental day and night. In other words, circadian factors decide whether we are diurnal or nocturnal. The seat of the circadian rhythms is suprachiasmatic nucleus as we shall see.

NEUROANATOMY OF SLEEP AND WAKEFULNESS

Wakefulness is maintained by the ascending reticular activating system, which is composed of mono-amine nuclei. It includes noradrenergic nuclei (locus ceruleus), cholinergic nuclei (lateral-dorsal tegmental nuclei and pedunculopontine nuclei), serotonergic nuclei (raphe nuclei), dopaminergic nuclei

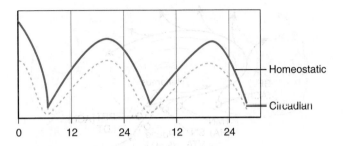

FIGURE 6.1.1

Homoeostatic and circadian regulation of sleep.

(ventral tegmental area) and histaminergic nuclei (tuberomamillary nuclei). These stimulate the cortical neurons and keep us awake and alert. Orexin neurons of hypothalamus modulate the activity of these neuronal groups. Activity of these neuronal groups is inhibited by the GABA neurons that are present in the ventrolateralpreoptic area (VLPO), and thus we fall asleep. This pathway is responsible for the homoeostatic regulation of sleep (Fig. 6.1.2).

Circadian regulation of sleep is regulated by the amount and intensity of light falling on the retina. This information is conveyed to suprachiasmatic nuclei (SCN) through retinohypothalamic tract. Absence of light stimulates the SCN and activates the pineal body to secrete melatonin through a pathway involving paraventricular nuclei and superior cervical ganglion. Melatonin receptors are present in many areas of the brain and they induce sleep. Detailed account of this mechanism is beyond the scope of this chapter.

Suprachiasmatic nuclei communicate with the VLPO and orexin neurons through the dorsomedial hypothalamic nucleus (Fig. 6.1.2). This shows that homoeostatic and circadian drives interact with each other to regulate sleep and wakefulness. State of sleep and wakefulness that we are in, depends upon the relative activity of sleep promoting factors and wake promoting factors, a mechanism known as flip-flop switch (Fig. 6.1.3).

MACRO-ARCHITECTURE OF SLEEP

Sleep is not a unitary phenomenon and it is divided into two major stages depending upon the elecrophysiological findings—non–rapid-eye-movement (NREM) sleep and rapid-eye-movement (REM) sleep. Both these stages keep alternating with a period of 90–120 min and thus, in a given night we have three to four such cycles (Fig. 6.1.4). REM sleep is predominantly dependent upon the circadian factors and thus, length of REM episode increases as the night progresses. On the other hand, homoeostatic sleep pressure regulates the 'slow wave sleep'; thus, it is seen in the first half of the night, when the sleep pressure is high.

NREM sleep makes 70–80% of the total sleep period. As we drift into sleep, we enter into stage 1 (N1 stage) and after spending few minutes in N1, stage 2 (N2) sleep appears (Fig. 6.1.5A). N2 sleep is characterized by sleep spindles and K-complexes (Fig. 6.1.5B). Deep sleep (also known as delta wave sleep or slow wave sleep or N3 sleep) is characterized by the presence of delta waves for more than 20% time in an epoch (Fig. 6.1.5C). Normally, among adults, N1 sleep accounts for 5% of the total sleep time; N2 between 40–50% and N3 sleep approximately 20% of the total sleep time.

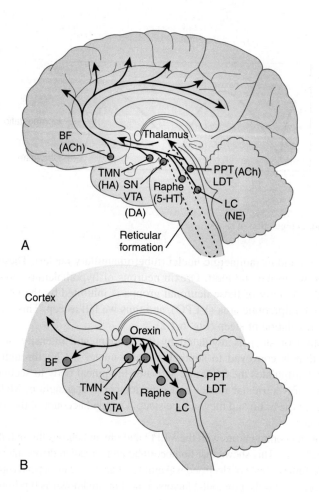

FIGURE 6.1.2

Neuroanatomy of sleep and wakefulness.

On the other hand, REM sleep is characterized by a low-voltage mixed frequency activity in the EEG, profound hypotonia in skeletal muscles and REMs. Around 20% of the total sleep time is spent in REM sleep among adults (Fig. 6.1.5D).

VIGNETTE

A 40-year-old woman presents with complaints of difficulty in falling asleep and nonrefreshing sleep for the past 3 years. She goes to bed at around 10 pm and it takes her approximately 60–90 min to fall asleep. She wakes up at 7 am but feels tired and often complains of morning headache.

She says that she has an urge to move her legs when she goes to bed and is relieved by doing so. This urge increases when she tries to lay still. She has never felt this urge during the day, even when she takes rest.

Her husband also gave history of night-time snoring, snorting and witnessed pauses in breath. She often talks during sleep and sometimes makes abnormal movements.

During the day, she feels sleepy and often falls asleep at odd places, eg, while watching the television, travelling in a car and while reading books. She often loses track while talking to people and she ascribes it to her daytime sleepiness.

She has hypertension and diabetes which are poorly controlled despite best of her efforts. Examination showed high-arched hard palate, large tongue and accumulation of submental fat. Central obesity is also visible. Her height is 165 cm and her weight is 105 Kg. Based on the history and examination, diagnosis of obstructive sleep apnoea hypopnoea syndrome (OSAHS) with restless legs syndrome (RLS) with systemic hypertension with type II diabetes mellitus was made and polysomnography was advised.

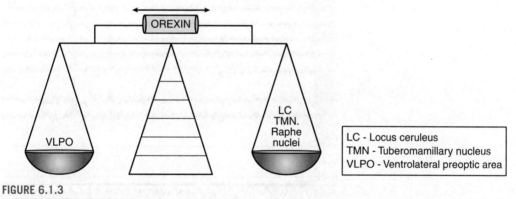

FIGURE 6.1.3

Flip-flop model for sleep regulation.

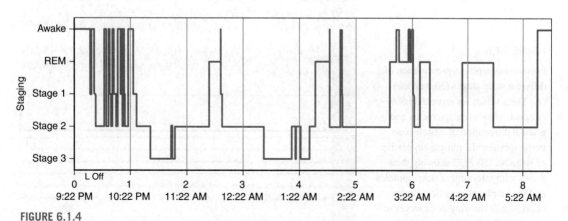

FIGURE 6.1.4

Normal hypnogram showing progression of sleep stages across night.

(Source: *Himalayan Hospital, Dehradun*)

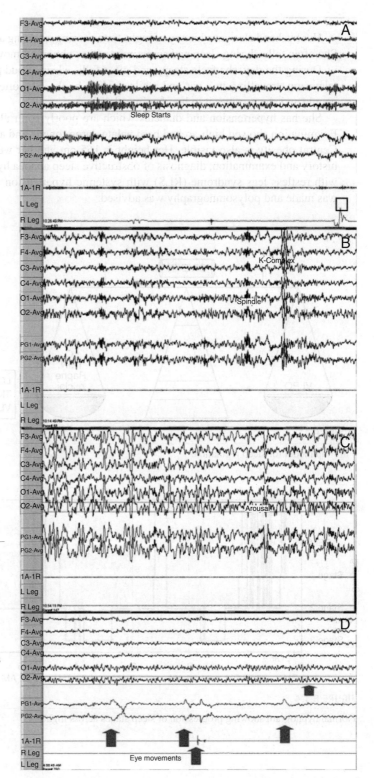

FIGURE 6.1.5

Polysomnographic representation of different sleep stages (30-s epoch). (A) Theta waves for more than 50% of epoch, slow eye movements and gradual diminution of muscle tone in the submentalis muscle suggestive of stage N1.(B) EEG showing theta waves with intermittent sleep spindles and K-complexes suggesting stage N2.(C) EEG showing delta waves in more than 20% of the epoch suggestive of stage N3.(D) EEG shows low-voltage mixed frequency activity, low tone in EMG and darting eye movements suggestive of REM sleep.

CLINICAL PICTURE

Clinical picture depends upon the type of disorder that we are dealing with. There are a number of sleep disorders; hence, we will briefly describe the disorders that are important for you as an undergraduate. With each of these disorders, we will briefly describe the pathophysiology as well as the management.

INSOMNIA

This is characterized by inability to fall asleep or multiple nocturnal awakenings or early morning awakening with difficulty in falling back asleep. These symptoms must be present despite good opportunities for sleep and must interfere with personal, social or occupational functioning. They should be present on at least three nights a week for a period of at least 3 months. This is termed as 'insomnia disorder' and if the duration of symptoms is less, the diagnosis is 'situational or acute insomnia'.

It develops due to an imbalance between sleep-promoting and wake-promoting mechanisms, as described above. It is seen in 10–15% of the population. Certain factors, eg, female gender, advancing age and persistent stress predispose to insomnia. If we do not treat situational insomnia, it converts into insomnia disorder. Many of us think that insomnia complaints seen in patients of anxiety and depression are the symptoms of those disorders. However, it must be remembered that insomnia is no longer considered merely as a symptom of psychiatric disorder; rather, if it persists long enough, it gets dissociated from the original disorder and starts running an independent course. Before making diagnosis of insomnia, you must rule out habitual short sleeping, narcolepsy, circadian rhythms sleep disorders, OSA, stimulant intoxication and, lastly, withdrawal of neurodepressive substances.

Situational insomnia can be managed with the help of hypnotics. A number of options are available for the treatment of situation insomnia—benzodiazepines (lorazepam 2 mg/day; clonazepam 0.5 mg/day), 'z' drugs (zolpidem 10 mg/day; eszopiclone 2 mg/day), sedating antihistaminics (promethazine 25 mg/day) and, lastly, sedating antidepressants (trazodon 50 mg/day; mirtazepine 15 mg/day). Depending upon the clinical conditions, drug interactions with the other medications thatpatient is taking and adverse effects, one of these medicines may be chosen.

However, insomnia disorder should be treated using cognitive behaviour therapy for insomnia (CBT-I) as this has been found to reduce the chances of relapse.

HYPERSOMNOLENCE DISORDER

This is characterized by excessive sleepiness despite 7 h of sleep during the main sleep period. This may present as repeated dozing or recurrent naps in a given day. These patients find it difficult to be alert after an abrupt awakening. Even when the main sleep period is extended beyond 9 h, they do not feel fresh. To be considered clinically significant, symptoms must be present at least thrice a week for at least 3 months.

It develops due to an imbalance between the sleep-promoting and wake-promoting mechanisms.It is seen with a prevalence of 1% and is seen between both genders with equal frequency. It can be idiopathic which starts during adolescence and often runs a chronic course. If it is recurrent, Klein–Levine syndrome (KLS) and recurrent hypersomnia of menstruation should be considered. Hypersomnia must be differentiated from narcolepsy, sleep apnoea, circadian rhythm sleep disorder, insufficient sleep syndrome and atypical depression in addition to substance abuse.

Night-time polysomnography reveals increased total sleep time and multiple sleep latency test (MSLT) shows short sleep-onset latency (less than 8 min). Wake-promoting drugs, eg, modafinil (50–100 mg/day), may be used to treat this condition.

NARCOLEPSY

It is characterized by recurrent irresistible urges to fall asleep or involuntary dozing in a given day. Like hypersomnolence disorder, symptoms must be present for at least three times a week for 3 months. In addition, cataplexy may be seen. Cataplexy is characterized by sudden loss of muscle tone in the presence of normal consciousness. This loss of muscle tone can vary in severity and in extent; in some cases, it may manifest just as a jaw drop or closure of eyelid, whereas in other cases, it may involve large muscles of the body and may lead to a fall. Hypnogogic (while drifting into sleep) and hypnopompic (while waking up) hallucinations may be seen. Patients describe these hallucination as, 'as if I was dreaming', 'a feeling of dreaming' or 'seeing some images' at the transition of sleep and wakefulness. In addition, some patients may report sleep paralysis. Sleep paralysis is a terrifying experience where a patient wakes up from sleep and feels that he/she is not able to breath and not able to move any of his/her body parts. After a few seconds, the patient regains the tone in his/her body. This experience is often ascribed to the witchcraft by one set of patients.

Its prevalence is between 0.02% and 0.04% with equal gender distribution. Usually it appears in children and adolescents. First symptom is usually hypersomnolence and cataplexy appears after a year in half of the cases.

This condition results from hypocretin dysfunction and hence often, but not always, the deficiency is seen (CSF hypocretin < 110 pg/mL). Deficient hypocretin is often associated with HLA DQB1*0602. Night-time polysomnography depicts sleep-onset REM (SOREMPs, ie, REM sleep appears within 15 min of sleep onset) and MSLT shows SOREMPs in at least two sleep periods with sleep latency less than 8 min.

Differential diagnosis includes sleep apnoea, circadian rhythm sleep disorder, insufficient sleep syndrome and depression, in addition to hypersomnolence disorder. Hypnogogic and hypnopompic hallucinations must be differentiated from schizophrenia and cataplexy from atonic seizures.

Treatment of narcolepsy is based on the target symptoms: for cataplexy, tricyclic antidepressants (eg, imipramine 10–25 mg/day) or selective serotonin reuptake inhibitors (eg, fluoxetine 20 mg/day) may be used as they abort *REM sleep atonia*; for hypersomnia, wake-promoting drugs (eg, modafinil 50–100 mg/day) and scheduled naps may be used. Recently, sodium oxybutate or gamma-hydroxy-butyrate (GHB) has been marketed, which has been found effective in managing all symptoms of narcolepsy.

RESTLESS LEGS SYNDROME

RLS is characterized by recurrent urge to move legs, especially at night, which may or may not be accompanied by abnormal sensation in calf muscles, eg, bubbling, worms crawling, tickling and dull aching. These symptoms worsen at rest and are relieved by moving the legs or application of counter-stimulation, eg, massaging, stretching or pressing the affected area. Rheumatoid arthritis, varicose veins, neuropathy, sciatica and exertional myalgia must be excluded before making the diagnosis.

Certain conditions predispose to develop RLS that include iron deficiency, pregnancy, chronic kidney disease and hypoxemic conditions. Population prevalence is around 4–5%. This disorder has female predisposition and have bimodel age of presentation—adolescence and another peak at around 40 years. At present, it is considered to be caused by deficiency of dopamine in the brain and hence, dopaminergic drugs (eg, levodopa) and dopamine agonists (eg, ropinirole 0.25–4 mg/day; pramipexole 0.125–1 mg/day) are prescribed to treat this condition.

SLEEP APNOEA

Sleep apnoea is defined as cessation of breathing for at least 10 s during sleep. Depending upon the effort for breathing, this can be divided into two types—obstructive sleep apnea (OSA) and central sleep apnoea (CSA) (Fig. 6.1.6).

Between both conditions, OSA is more common with a population prevalence of around 5–8%; hence, here we will restrict our discussion to OSA. Certain factors, eg, male gender, retrognathia, retrusion of maxilla, adenotonsillar enlargement andmacroglossia, predispose to this condition by *narrowing the upper airway mechanically*; sedative hypnotics, alcohol, etc. can reduce the pharyngeal dilator muscle tone exert the same effect by *neural mechanisms*. Obesity increases the thickness of parapharyngeal pads of fat that push the pharyngeal muscles inwards to reduce the calibre of upper airway.

Common symptoms of OSA include snoring, snorting, witnessed pauses in breath during sleep, poor quality sleep, recurrent arousals because of chocking sensations, nocturia, sleep talking, sleep walking, excessive daytime sleepiness, memory lapses, morning headache and fatigue.

Diagnosis is usually made by overnight diagnostic polysomnography. This must be differentiated from depression, somatoform disorders, hypersomnolence disorder and narcolepsy to name a few. Treatment depends upon the severity of the condition and comorbidities. Mild OSA is usually managed by positional therapy, weight control and lifestyle modification. On the other hand, positive airway pressure (PAP) therapy may be required to treat moderate to severe OSA. Depending upon the comorbidities, patient may require craniofacial or palatopharyngeal or bariatric surgery.

Treatment must be instituted energetically as untreated OSA can lead to hypertension, coronary artery disease, metabolic syndrome, diabetes mellitus and stroke, besides cardiac arrhythmia.

CIRCADIAN RHYTHM SLEEP DISORDERS

These are those conditions that arise because of the mismatch between circadian time and environmental time. This leads to dissociation between homoeostatic and circadian drives of sleep and thus leads to one of the following conditions: inability to fall asleep; difficulty in waking up at desired time, poor quality sleep or excessive sleep. These conditions interfere with the daily functioning and thus are the focus of concern. Table 6.1.1 describes common circadian rhythm sleep disorders.

These disorders are treated by the chronotherapy (rescheduling sleep) and timed exposure to bright light therapy. Melatonin (3 mg/day) and its agonists (eg, ramelteon 8–16 mg/day) may be tried to reset the circadian rhythm.

PARASOMNIA

Parasomniais characterized by abnormal movements during sleep that are expected during normal sleep, eg, sleep walking and sleep talking. These disorders may be classified further depending upon the sleep stage, ie, NREM sleep and REM sleep (Table 6.1.2).

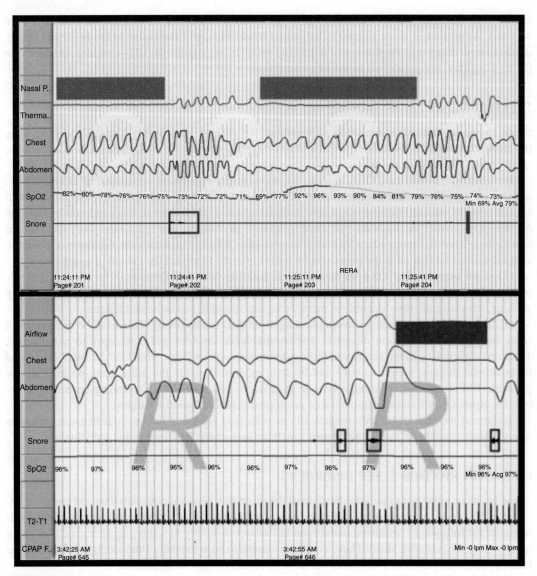

FIGURE 6.1.6

Epochs showing OSA and CSA (120-s epoch). Upper part of the figure shows absence of airflow (nasal P) for more than 10 s along with paradoxical movements of chest and abdomen and oxygen desaturation (SpO$_2$) during N2 sleep (see 2 in the background) suggestive of OSA. Lower part of the figure depicts cessation of airflow, chest and abdominal movements for more than 10 s suggestive of CSA.

(Source: *Himalayan Hospital, Dehradun*)

Table 6.1.1 Circadian Rhythm Sleep Disorders

	Advance Sleep Wake Phase Disorder	Delayed Sleep Wake Phase Disorder	Irregular Sleep Wake Type	Shift Worker Disorder
Prevalence	1% in middle aged	0.17% in population, but 7% among adolescents	Unknown	5–10% of night workers
Age of onset	Common in old age	Usually adolescence	Variable	Variable, depends upon the exposure to the shift work
Predisposing factors	1. Reduced light exposure in evening and light exposure during morning 2. PER2 gene mutation	1. Longer circadian period 2. Hypersensitivity to evening light 3. Mutation in PER3 gene	Neurodevelopmental and neurodegenerative disorders	Morning chronotype and long sleepers
Presentation	Sleeping earlier than desired bedtime, usually at least 2 h earlier and waking up early in the morning with adequate total sleep time	Sleeping late at night and waking up late in the morning	Sleep and wake period during day and night are fragmented	Are not able to maintain alertness on job and fall asleep when off-work due to misaligned and variable time for sleep

Table 6.1.2 Parasomnias

	NREM sleep: *Usually appear in the first half of the night (see sleep macro-architecture)*					REM sleep: *Usually during second half of the night*	
	Sleep Walking	**Sleep Talking**	**Sleep-Related Eating Disorder**	**Sexsomnia**	**Sleep Terrors**	**Nightmare Disorder**	**Rem Sleep Behaviour Disorder**
Age of onset	Childhood	Childhood	Adolescence	Adolescence and adults	Childhood	Childhood	Elderly
Prevalence	2–3% among children	1–5%	Not known	Not known	Not known	Variable but increases with the progression of age till adulthood	0.5% in general population
Predisposing factors	1. Sleep deprivation, fatigue, sleep–wake schedule disruption, hypnotic use, alcohol withdrawal, stress, fever and sleep fragmentation often associated with sleep apnoea and restless legs syndrome, especially in adults 2. Genetic factors are more common in those with positive family history						Neurodegenerative disorders and antidepressants
Clinical presentation	Walking during sleep usually with blank face and open eyes, difficulty in waking up, no recall of the episode	Talks during sleep, often coherent and able to communicate but not able to recall after waking up; no recall of the episode	Eating during sleep, often large amounts and not able to recall in the morning and when made to wake up	Sexual activity during sleep, often violent but not able to recall after being woken up, difficult to wake up	Sudden onset inconsolable crying during sleep, appears frightened, not able to appreciate the surroundings and not able to recall the episode or dream after waking up	Frightening dreams that wake up the person having sympathetic arousal, but becomes oriented soon after waking up, able to recall the dream	These patients often act in their dreams, often the dreams are violent and hence they injure themselves or their bed partner; they are able to recall the dream on waking up

Level 1 polysomnography may help to pick sleep disorders. In REM sleep behaviour disorder, normally occurring atonia during REM sleep is absent, thus patients are left to enact their dreams (they act what they dream). They must be differentiated from sleep-related seizures. Taking care of predisposing factors treats them. Benzodiazepines may be used to treat NREM parasomnias. Clonazepam (0.5–2 mg/day) is effective in REM sleep behaviour disorder.

SUMMARY

- Sleep disorders are common in general population.
- Sleeplessness or poor-quality sleep does not always indicate insomnia.
- Diagnosis of sleep disorders is of paramount importance as they are treatable.
- Untreated sleep disorders are a health hazard and often run a chronic course.
- Overnight video synchronized attended polysomnography with manual scoring of data is gold standard for the diagnosis of sleep disorders.

FURTHER READING

1. American Academy of Sleep Medicine. (2014). "The International Classification of Sleep Disorders, Third Edition (ICSD-3)." Author, Darian, IL.
2. Berry R. B., Brooks R., Gamaldo C. E., Harding S. M., Lloyd R. M., Marcus C. L., and Vaughn B. V. for the American Academy of Sleep Medicine. (2015). "The AASM Manual for the Scoring of Sleep and Associated Events: Rules, Terminology and Technical Specifications, version 2.2 www.aasmnet.org." American Academy of Sleep Medicine, Darien, IL.

HEADACHES IN PSYCHIATRY PRACTICE

7.1

Ravi Gupta

In psychiatry practice it is not uncommon to find patients with headache. It has been reported that nearly 70% of the patients with chronic migraine and chronic tension-type headache have some or the other psychiatric disorder. You must already be knowing that headaches can be classified into two major groups—primary and secondary.

Primary headaches are diagnosed where in a patient with headache, we do not find any abnormality in the structural neuroimaging, eg, CT scan or MRI of the brain and all other causes of secondary headaches, eg, ocular causes, otorhinolaryngological reasons, systemic causes, inflammation, dental pathologies, substance use disorder and trauma have been excluded. Thus, we can say that primary headaches are similar to psychiatric disorders, where you do not find any pathology on the routine investigations.

Moreover, although some of the primary headaches are commonly seen with psychiatric disorders (as we have mentioned earlier), a number of psychiatric disorders themselves have headache as a symptom, eg, somatic symptoms disorder, functional neurological symptoms disorder, depression and drug intoxication or withdrawal to name a few. Headaches associated with psychiatric disorders have been kept in the Appendix in the International Classification of Headache Disorders 3rd edition (ICHD-3). This also necessitates the need for in-depth understanding of headache by the psychiatrists.

In this chapter, we will focus on commonly encountered primary headaches due to limitation of space. If you are interested in headache medicine, you may refer to any of the textbooks dedicated to this specialty. We are omitting the taxonomy part here, because it is best to follow ICHD-3 for the classification of headaches.

VIGNETTE

A 30-year-old woman presented with recurrent headaches since past 6 months. She mentioned that headache started around 15 years back, but has increased in frequency during past 6 months. Since past 6 months she has been experiencing two to three episodes of severe headache, each lasting 10–12 h almost once a week. However, she has never been headache free during this period and a dull ache persisted all the time. She reported that during dull pain she has felt 'as if a band is tied around her head' and this headache often did not interfere with her daily activities. She did not report any other symptom associated with dull pain. On the other hand, severe headache usually starts at temple and she experiences the pain in the ipsilateral neck at that time. Pain is severe and pulsating in nature. She complains of nausea and/or vomiting with this headache. She reports that during the period of headache, noise appears louder (phonophobia) and lights brighter (photophobia). Hence, she prefers to lie down in a calm and dark room. She denied experiencing any aura. It lasts for 10–12 h if she is not able to take rest. If she takes rest (usually for 4–5 h), then it subsides by the time she wakes up. If somebody wakes her up during this period, the headache increases in severity and then lasts for 2–3 days. Simple analgesics help her to get rid of the headache. Based on the history, diagnosis of chronic tension-type headache with migraine without aura was made.

NEUROBIOLOGY OF HEADACHE

In the prodromal period, an individual feels the initial signs of headache. However, not all prodromes develop into headache. This is explained in Fig. 7.1.1 in detail.

In some of the cases, prodrome sets in the sensitization of trigeminal neurons, which can either be peripheral or can be central. *Peripheral sensitization* occurs when the neurons in close proximity to the dural vessels start reacting to the release of the inflammatory markers around the blood vessels. It takes around 10 min to develop and is clinically manifested by throbbing headache and increase in pain intensity in response to the activities that increase the intracranial pressure, eg, bending forward or coughing. *Central sensitization* of the trigeminal and thalamic neurons induces allodynia in scalp and body, respectively. Thus, patients with migraine often do not like any pressure on their face, scalp and body. Thus, they remove tight spectacles, headbands or hat, tight cloths and do not like to be hugged or massaged. It takes around 2 h to develop trigeminal sensitization and around 4 h to develop thalamic sensitization.

Molecules acting on the sites of peripheral sensitization, eg, calcitonin gene related peptide (CGRP) antibodies, can prevent peripheral and thereafter central sensitization and prevent the development of migraine attack. However, drugs like triptans that act on $5HT_{1B}/_{1D}$ receptors act at the junction of peripheral and central neurons (dorsal horn) in trigeminal nucleus to prevent central sensitization and thus abort the migraine attack, provided they are given before the symptoms of allodynia develop. Moreover, ergots act at the level of trigeminal nucleus and thus they are effective even after the central sensitization sets in.

Neurobiology of other headaches (eg, tension-type headache, cluster headache) is thought to overlap the pathophysiology of migraine. However, their detailed description is out of the scope of this book.

CLINICAL PICTURE

Clinical picture varies from one to another headache. Migraine typically presents as unilateral severe throbbing-type of headache that is most commonly located over the temporal region. This headache lasts for 4–72 h and often associated with nausea and/or vomiting. These patients feel sounds as loud (phonophobia) and light as more intense (photophobia) during the migraine attack. Estimation of the duration of headache is important in these cases, eg, suppose an individual falls asleep after 1 h of developing migraine attack and wakes up after 5 h feeling free of pain, then the time spent in sleep must

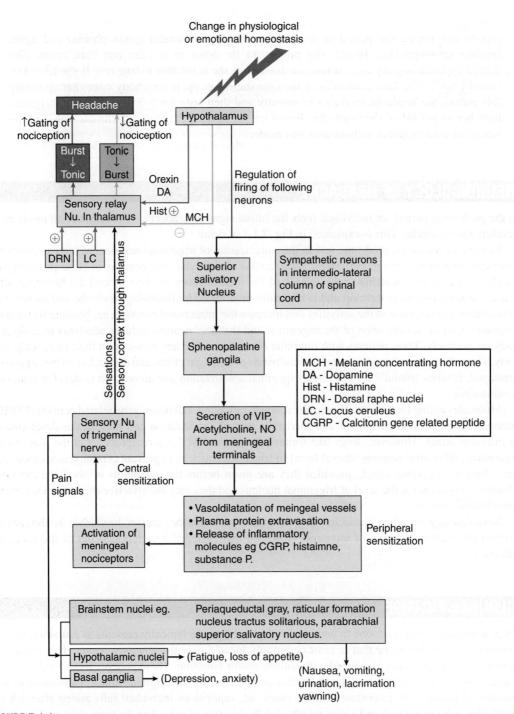

FIGURE 7.1.1

Neurobiology of migraine.

be included in the duration of headache. Some patients have associated aura that is most commonly visual—a fortification spectra or shimmering lights that are superimposed upon the normal background visible from the eye. Sometimes, these patients may have gustatory or olfactory aura, although they are less common. Based on the presence of aura, migraine may be divided into two subtypes—migraine without aura and migraine with aura. Chronic migraine is diagnosed when the patient complains of migraine more than 15 days a month for at least 3 months.

Migraine has multiple triggering factors that include alteration in the timing, duration or quality of sleep, hunger or delaying the meals, change in the atmosphere, humidity, heat, extreme cold, strong smells and emotional stress. Similarly, besides medicines, a number of factors can relieve migraine, eg, falling asleep.

Tension-type headache is a dull aching headache that is appreciated as a 'band tied around head'. It can last from 30 min to 7 days and may be accompanied by either phonophobia or photophobia, but never both. When it occurs for less than 15 days a month, it is called episodic tension-type headache and if it occurs more than 15 days a month for at least 3 months, it is called chronic tension-type headache.

Cluster headache is a severe pain localized to the orbit, supraorbital region or to the temporal region and it is accompanied by a sense of agitation. It can last from 15 min to 3 h. This is accompanied by ipsilateral autonomic symptoms that appear due to trigeminofacial connection and present as at least one of the following: reddening of eye, lacrimation, eyelid oedema, miosisorptosis, nasal blockade or rhinorrhoea, sweating or flushing over ipsilateral forehead and face and sense of fullness in the ear. The frequency of attacks varies from one every other day to more than eight episodes a day. This disease has a pain-free interval that can vary between months to years. When untreated cluster headache is present for less than a year and two cluster periods have an interval longer than 1 month, it is known as episodic cluster headache. Chronic cluster headache is diagnosed when the disease is present for more than year without remission for at least 1 month.

Medication overuse headache develops when someone overuses analgesics, triptans, ergots and opioids. This headache lasts for more than 15 days in a month. In addition there is history of regular intake of pain-relieving drugs for at least 3 months. Regular intake of pain-relieving medication is defined based on the class of the drugs. Regular use of analgesics is considered when they are taken for more than 15 days in a month during the symptomatic period; for ergots, triptans and opioids, regular use is defined as use of the medications for more than 10 days in a month.

DIFFERENTIAL DIAGNOSIS

These headaches must be differentiated from other primary headaches that arise from the craniofacial pathologies and from one another. They must be differentiated from headache arising due to intoxication or withdrawal of substances of abuse, eg, alcohol or opioids and medication overuse headache and all of the secondary headaches.

MANAGEMENT

Precipitating factors must be avoided and use of relieving factors must be promoted. For migraine and tension-type headache, simple analgesics (eg, paracetamol), combined analgesics (eg, paracetamol with ibuprofen) or opioids (eg, propoxyphene) may be used as abortificants. Triptans (eg, sumatriptan 50 mg) and ergots (eg, dihydroergotamine 0.5 mg) can abort migraine and cluster headache.

Prophylactic therapy for the tension-type headache includes use of antidepressants (eg, sertraline 25–50 mg/day; amitriptyline 10–75 mg/day). Propranolol (10–160 mg/day) can be used for prophylaxis of migraine. Valproate (250–1000 mg/day) is effective for prophylaxis of migraine, cluster headache and medication overuse headache.

SUMMARY

- Headaches are common in psychiatry practice.
- Primary headaches are frequently comorbid with psychiatric disorders.
- Tension type headache is the most common type of headache, although in clinics, migraine is the most common type of headache.
- Adequate diagnosis and management of headache is important for complete remission of psychiatric morbidity.

FURTHER READING

1. Burnstein R., Noseda R., and Borsook D. (2015). Migraine: Multiple Processes, Complex Pathophysiology. *The Journal of Neuroscience,* 35:6619–6629.
2. Hcadache Classification Committee of International Headache Society (2013). International Classification of Headache Disorders, 3rd Edition. *Cephalalgia,* 33:629–808.

EMERGENCY CONDITIONS IN PSYCHIATRY

8.1

Ravi Gupta

Like any other medical branch, emergencies are not uncommon in psychiatry. Common emergency situations that you will come across during your practice may be related to the disease or may be related to the treatment. They are outlined in Table 8.1.1. If left unattended, they may lead to a major complication or loss of life of the patient and, in case of agitated patients, injury to self or harm to others.

In this chapter we will discuss regarding suicide, prolonged fasting related to psychiatric disorder, agitated patients and catatonia. Intoxication or withdrawal of a substance of abuse and delirium have been discussed in detail in the chapters on substance-related disorders (Chapter 4.1) and neurocognitive disorders (Chapter 5.1), respectively. Similarly, emergencies arising out of psychotropic treatment are discussed in the chapter on psychopharmacology (Chapter 10.1).

SELF-INFLICTED INJURY

Self-harm is not an uncommon condition and, as a medical practitioner, you will see many of the cases that after inflicting any injury to themselves show in emergency departments with various complications.

NOSOLOGY

DSM-5 does not include it as a psychiatric disorder but recognizes it as a condition that requires further study. DSM-5 categorizes self-harm into two entities—suicidal behaviour disorder and non-suicidal

Table 8.1.1 Emergency Conditions in Psychiatry	
Disease related	1. Self-inflicted injury 2. Intoxication or withdrawal of substances of abuse 3. Delirium 4. Patients presenting with prolonged fasting related to eating disorders, schizophrenia or depression 5. Agitated patient 6. Catatonia
Treatment related	1. Drug-related dystonia 2. Neuroleptic malignant syndrome 3. Lithium toxicity 4. Overdose of medication

self-injury. Thus, it clarifies that *all self-inflicted injuries are not suicide attempts*. Similar to DSM-5, ICD-10 also does not include it in the category of psychiatric disorders and mentions it with the name of intentional self-harm under the section on external causes of morbidity and mortality (categories X60 to X84).

VIGNETTE

A 30-year-old man was brought to the emergency room in unconscious state. Clinical information disclosed a history of self-hanging approximately 2 h back. He was noticed hanging from the fan by his mother, who called other members of the family for help. There was no history of any psychiatric illness, chronic illness related to the patient or of the family members. The family members did not find any suicide note in their home. According to the mother, apparently he was well 3 h back, when he had an altercation with his brother. After this, his brother left home and he went to his room. There was no history of any psychiatric illness or similar attempts in the past. Family history was also negative for self-harm and psychiatric disorders.

Medical examination showed that vitals were stable but he was in the state of delirium. He was maintaining 97% oxygen saturation on room air. Pupils were normal sized and normally reacting on both sides. Glasgow coma scale score was E2M2V4. Neck showed a ligature mark (Fig. 8.1.1).

Further neurological examination and mental status examination could not be performed. Drug abuse screening test was negative. MRI scan of the brain and cervical spine was ordered. Based on the history and examination, diagnosis of suicidal behaviour disorder was made.

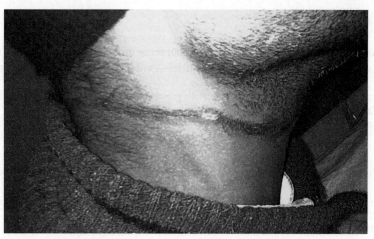

FIGURE 8.1.1

Strangulation mark of hanging on a patient.

(Source: *Himalayan Hospital, Dehradun*)

CLINICAL PICTURE

Suicidal behaviour disorder can be diagnosed when during the previous 2 years a person had inflicted an injury upon him/her or committed any other act that was expected to lead to loss of life at the time of commencement. However, this act should not have occurred during delirium or intoxication and not for the political and religious objectives. It means that religious practices like 'samadhi' among Hindus and 'santhaaraa' among Jains cannot be considered suicidal behavioural disorder. It must be noted that having suicidal ideation or preparatory acts should not be considered as suicidal behaviour disorder. Depending upon the type of method chosen, it may be classified into violent, eg, jumping, hanging, shooting oneself, or nonviolent, eg, ingestion of pills or poisonous substances.

Another method of classifying the suicide depends upon the degree of planning—it may either be a premeditated act or an impulsive act. In the premeditated act, a person often starts preparing for the act days or weeks ahead. Before committing the act, he/she makes a firm plan to commit the act, writes a suicide note, try to manage all the responsibilities so that his/her family members do not face any trouble afterwards. Many such patients often disclose it to their friends or family members by some or the other means or sometimes make just a passing remark during a routine conversation. Thus, it is advised that these kinds of remarks should be taken seriously. On the other hand, impulsive acts are committed during the period of frustration by the person harbouring high impulsivity. These people often do not want to end their life, but during periods of frustration, they are not able to tolerate it and commit these kinds of acts. Common examples of impulsive suicide acts include committing this act after being forbidden to purchase a gadget or after failing in an examination or after an altercation in family. Lastly, suicide can be differentiated upon the basis of lethality. Lethal attempts require prolonged hospitalization, whereas those of low lethality require just an emergency visit.

A comparison of disorders related to self-inflicted injury has been made in Table 8.1.2.

Table 8.1.2 Comparison of Disorders Related to Self-Inflicted Injury (DSM-5)

Factors	Suicidal Behaviour Disorder	Nonsuicidal Self-Injury
Duration and frequency	At least once in the past 2 years	Five or more days in the past 1 year
Suicidal intent	Present	Absent
Motive	End of life	1. To relieve negative emotional or cognitive states 2. To resolve relational trouble 3. To induce positive emotions At least one of the following should be present: 1. Negative emotions just before the act 2. Difficult to control the recurring thought of harming oneself before the act 3. Frequent thoughts of inflicting self-injury

NEUROBIOLOGY

The neurobiological understanding of this disorder is limited by the fact that functional neuroimaging is not possible before or during the act. However, post-mortem brain studies, CSF studies and blood studies show that it is associated with high 5-hydroxy indole acetic acid (5-HIAA), a metabolite of serotonin and increment in $5HT_{2A}$ receptors on platelets. These are markers for the impulsivity and these persons harbour a trait for high impulsivity (please refer to Chapter 3.8). Stress can precipitate the act in these persons, which can be assessed using hypothalamic–pituitary–adrenal axis dysfunction (assessed using dexamethasone suppression test) and concentration of brain-derived neurotropic factor (BDNF) in cerebrospinal fluid.

EPIDEMIOLOGY AND RISK FACTORS

It is uncommon among children but it has been reported through adolescence. Some of the factors increase the risk of suicide, eg, chronic nontreatable medical and surgical disorders; psychiatric disorders, eg, mood disorders, schizophrenia, alcohol-use disorder, borderline personality disorder, antisocial personality disorder, eating disorders, adjustment disorders; and, lastly, history of a well-planned, but failed attempt. Thus, these patients should be regularly screened for the risk of suicide attempt. It is a common belief that by questioning a person for suicidal ideas and plans, you are sowing a seed in his/her mind to commit it. On the contrary, screening the patient for the risk of suicide actually encourages the patient to share his/her problems (thoughts or previous attempts of the suicidal acts) and thus the risk may be reduced.

Factors adding to the risk of recurrent suicide attempts have been listed in Table 8.1.3.

MANAGEMENT

After a failed attempt, immediate management rests on the physicians and surgeons, depending upon the complication that the patient had presented with. Once the patient recovers and is able to communicate coherently, he/she must be assessed to rule out associated psychiatric and medical disorders, including other issues that lead to commencement of the act. Other conditions that had contributed in the attempt must be addressed. Psychiatric disorder should be addressed urgently using adequate measures; preferably using modified electroconvulsive therapy (mECT). Pharmacotherapy for the comorbid psychiatric disorder may be initiated as and when required and choice of medication depends upon the underlying illness. Nonpharmacological methods, eg, interpersonal therapy and family therapy may be used in case of interpersonal difficulties.

COURSE AND PROGNOSIS

It must be remembered that nearly one-fourth of the patients who attempt suicide, attempt it again. Some factors make them prone to/high risk for recurrence of attempts. These factors must be assessed while examining the patient. Thus, every attempt should be taken seriously and evaluated for the risk of future attempts.

Table 8.1.3 Factors Adding to the Risk of Recurrent Suicide Attempts
1. A premeditated attempt
2. Prior history of suicide attempts
3. Family history of suicide attempts
4. Personal or family history of psychiatric disorders
5. History of chronic untreatable disorders
6. Recent loss and feelings of ineptness
7. Poor social support
8. Substance abuse

PATIENTS PRESENTING WITH PROLONGED FASTING RELATED TO PSYCHIATRIC DISORDERS

Patients having some of the psychiatric disorders may present with prolonged fasting, eg, a patient with paranoid delusions may not eat anything because he/she believes that his/her food has been poisoned; depression may be associated with loss of appetite to the extent that the sufferer do not eat anything for days; and similarly, patients of anorexia nervosa may not eat anything or may be engaged in life-threatening dietary restrictions in an attempt to lose weight. These patients may present with a number of complications that are related to insufficiency of calories, deficiency of vitamins, minerals and, lastly, hypovolumia. Thus, they may be in a state of acute kidney injury and hypotension along with cardiac arrhythmias.

After prolonged fasting, when the food intake is initiated, these patients are at the risk of refeeding syndrome, which requires careful monitoring of food and calorie intake. In these patients, it is pertinent to address the condition in close association with a physician and a dietician. For detailed description of refeeding syndrome, you may refer to a textbook of medicine.

AGITATED PATIENTS

Although with the advent of effective drugs, agitated patients are seen less and less, yet it is a condition where you may be asked to attend and provide care. Among psychiatric disorders, aggression may be associated with schizophrenia, bipolar disorder, antisocial personality disorder, substance intoxication or withdrawal, excited catatonia and delirium. It is important that the underlying factors are ascertained and addressed.

Environmental stimuli may precipitate an episode of aggression and thus the environmental stimuli be reduced by keeping them in an isolated area. Pharmacologically, acute situation may be controlled using the antipsychotics, eg, haloperidol (5 mg every 30 min till the patient is sedated; however, lower dose should be used in patients with delirium), and benzodiazepine, eg, lorazepam (2 mg every 30 min till the patient is sedated). Some patients may require mECT for faster action.

CATATONIA

Catatonia is defined as a state where the psychomotor activity of the patient is either grossly reduced, sometimes to the extent of stupor or contrarily, patient may present with nongoal-directed excessive motor activity, which is independent of any external influence. Excited patients may appear aggressive.

NOSOLOGY

DSM-5 recognized catatonia as a separate entity and provides specifiers, eg, catatonia associated with another mental disorder; associated with another medical condition and, lastly, unspecified type. On the other hand, ICD-10 has included catatonia as a subtype of schizophrenia.

VIGNETTE

A 30-year-old male was brought to the emergency room with the complaints that he does not make any movement, spends a lot of time in one posture, does not talk to the people, does not follow any command and when spoken to, repeats what is said to him. These symptoms developed 20 days back. He does not have any history of substance abuse or any other neurological or medical disorder. However, he has a history of recurrent depressive episodes in the past. Vitals were stable. Neurological examination revealed rigidity throughout movements in all limbs. Mental status examination revealed posturing, psychogenic pillow and waxy flexibility. Based on the history and examination, diagnosis of catatonia associated with major depressive disorder: recurrent episodes, current episode major depressive disorder was made.

CLINICAL PICTURE

These patients present with a number of features that suggest a change in the psychomotor activity. Here, the word psychomotor suggests that in these patients, motor cortex and pyramidal tract are functioning normally; however, the problem lies at the will (psyche) to produce any movement.

When the activity is extremely reduced, patient may become stuperose, ie, do not make any motor activity even in an environment that is full of stimuli. In catalepsy, limbs are rigid and remain in the position in which they are *placed* by the examiner. In other words, they maintain the odd postures in which they are placed for the prolonged periods (eg, psychogenic pillow, where patients head is lifted from the bed to a significant extent and they maintain the same posture for a long period) despite instructing them that they are free to assume a comfortable posture. Many patients show posturing, ie, they maintain one posture for prolonged period that has been assumed *spontaneously*. Mutism is depicted as absence of verbal communication despite normal speech circuitry and resistance to external commands or not following commands represents negativism in catatonia. Patients who have waxy flexibility do not resist the movements of their body parts made by the examiner and it appears as if their body is made up of wax, which can be moulded into any shape without any resistance offered by the patient. All these symptoms are also known as negative symptoms.

When the psychomotor activity is increased, it may lead to non–goal-directed agitation. Another feature, stereotypy is characterized by repeating a movement without any reason that is not goal directed. On the contrary, patients showing mannerism repeatedly make a movement that signifies a specific purpose, but in the given situation, it is out of context, eg, saluting. Patients may also show grimacing, echolalia (repeating what is said to them instead of responding to it) and, lastly, echopraxia (imitating the examiner's movements).

NEUROBIOLOGY

Neurobiology of catatonia is not thoroughly known as a syndrome; however, with the current understanding we are able to explain its different symptoms. Stupor is related to the deficiency of dopamine in striatum leading to dominance of direct loop (1) over indirect corticio-striato-thalamo-cortical loop and (2) ultimately presenting as profound akinesia (stupor).

Initiation of movement at will require orbitofrontal cortex (OFC), dorsolateral prefrontal cortex and anterior cingulate gyrus that are connected to the motor cortex. Either OFC is dysfunctional in stupor or the connection between the orbitofrontal to motor and supplementary motor cortex is disrupted in catatonia, leading to akinesia seen across variety of symptoms (negativism and mutism). Poor activity in OFC leads to the shift of activity towards medical prefrontal cortex (that regulates social cognition; please refer to Chapter 2.4) and anterior cingulate gyrus. Anterior cingulate cortex has three distinct areas, ie, motor, cognitive and affective. Activity in each of these areas inhibits the remaining two areas. Thus, shifting of activity to affective area leads to inhibition of cognitive and motor areas of anterior cingulate gyrus along with compromise in ability to perceive movements and emotional state of others. The outcome appears as stupor and mutism.

Negativism, echopraxia, echolalia, stereotypy and perseveration are seen owing to disturbances in planning and monitoring of the new movement. OFC has the connection with ventrolateral prefrontal cortex (VLPFC), which is important for the monitoring of complex behaviour. This exerts negative control over the dorsolateral prefrontal cortex (DLPFC) that helps in planning the complex behaviour via reciprocal connections. Both these areas have reciprocal connections with posterior parietal cortex that is important for the recognition of movement in space. Poor activity in OFC, leads to poor inhibition of DLPFC by the VLPFC. Thus, any movement once started, keeps recurring resulting in stereotypy and mannerism. Due to dysfunctional DLPFC, patient is not able to plan new movement, resulting in imitation of other's movements or words leading to echopraxia and echolalia.

Posturing is considered to be related to the abnormality of right parietal cortex that is instrumental in providing the information regarding the visuospatial position of the body and limbs. It also provides inputs to terminate the movement, once the limb reaches in correct position. Posturing and catalepsy is associated with abnormal functioning of this area, leading to maintenance of a posture. (Fig. 8.1.2)

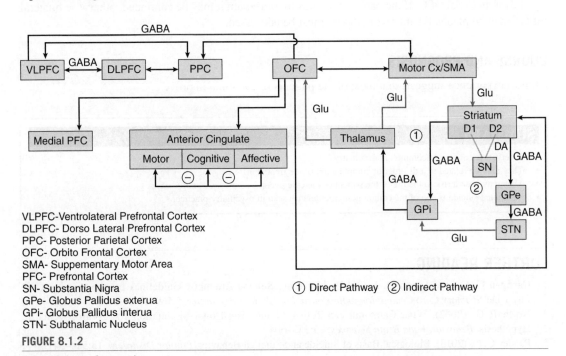

VLPFC-Ventrolateral Prefrontal Cortex
DLPFC- Dorso Lateral Prefrontal Cortex
PPC- Posterior Parietal Cortex
OFC- Orbito Frontal Cortex
SMA- Supplementary Motor Area
PFC- Prefrontal Cortex
SN- Substantia Nigra
GPe- Globus Pallidus exterua
GPi- Globus Pallidus interua
STN- Subthalamic Nucleus

FIGURE 8.1.2

Neurobiology of catatonia.

Waxy flexibility represents the hypertonia that maintains throughout the movement. This results from the downregulation of D2 receptors due to two different reasons—as we have already discussed, poor communication between OFC and motor cortex and, secondly, modulation of striatal D2 receptors by orbitofrontocortical loop.

Thus, we have seen that more than one area of the brain is instrumental in producing one symptom of catatonia. At the same time, one area is regulating more than one symptom. OFC has GABA-A receptors in high density to modulate activity in other areas. Dysfunction of OFC means that GABA-A receptors are dysfunctional. This is the reason that benzodiazepines and antipsychotics are effective in treatment of catatonia.

It must be noted that all the symptoms may not appear in a given patient. It is thus, best be considered as a syndrome where some of the areas in a given patient may go dysfunctional.

EPIDEMIOLOGY AND RISK FACTORS

Epidemiology is not known. Catatonia may be associated with a number of psychiatric conditions—schizophrenia, depression, mania and neurodevelopmental disorders. It may also be associated with some medical disorders, eg, hepatic encephalopathy and third ventricular tumour. Identification of underlying pathology is of paramount importance in planning the management.

MANAGEMENT

First line of management is lorazepam (2–12 mg/day) which acts on GABA. This may restore the activity of dysfunctional OFC. If the patient responds to lorazepam it may be continued, otherwise bilateral mECT may be planned. Underlying illness must be addressed.

COURSE AND PROGNOSIS

Clinical experience suggests that most of the patients of catatonia improve.

SUMMARY

- Emergencies are not uncommon in psychiatry.
- They may be related to a disorder or complication of the treatment.
- They may pose a risk to the life of the patient or the caregivers.
- Attempted suicide is one of the commonest emergencies seen in psychiatry practice.

FURTHER READING

1. Carrigan C. G., and Lynch D. J. (2003). Managing Suicide Attempts: Guidelines for the Primary Care Physician. *Primary Care Companion to the Journal of Clinical Psychiatry*, 5:169–174.
2. Northoff G. (2002). What Catatonia can Tellus About "Top-Down Modulation": A Neuropsychiatric Hypothesis. *Behavioral and Brain Sciences*, 25:555–604.
3. Pandey G. N. (2013). Biological Basis of Suicide and Suicidal Behavior. *Bipolar Disorders*, 15:524–541.

BEHAVIOURAL AND ELECTRICAL THERAPIES THAT AFFECT BRAIN FUNCTION

9.1

Ravi Gupta

Nonpharmacological therapies are those behavioural and cognitive techniques that are used to shape the behaviour and remove cognitive distortions in patients without using pharmacotherapeutic agents. This heading also includes some other techniques that use the methods that are different from pharmacotherapy and it includes electroconvulsive therapy (ECT) and repeated transcranial magnetic stimulation (r-TMS). Scope of behavioural therapies is not limited to psychiatry and they are useful in other branches of medical science as well! However, they have been studied best in psychiatric disorders because of behavioural manifestations of their symptoms.

PSYCHOTHERAPY AND BEHAVIOURAL THERAPIES

Psychotherapy aims to bring out a permanent change in personality by substituting the dysfunctional beliefs and behaviours. On the other hand, behaviour therapies have limited scope and they aim to delearn a maladaptive behaviour and substitute it with a context-specific acceptable behaviour. It must be remembered that these techniques are *not psychological* as they are often considered; rather they produce functional as well as structural changes in the brain, because they are based on the principles of learning (Fig. 9.1.1).

BASIC INFORMATION REGARDING BEHAVIOURAL TECHNIQUES

During these techniques, patient is encouraged to unlearn the dysfunctional belief or behaviour and to learn the rationale belief or acceptable behaviour. Thus, like pharmacotherapy, they have their own adverse effects and in the hands of an untrained person they may produce a deleterious effect on the patient's behaviour. This also signifies that one must have adequate training and experience while using these techniques. Just imagine, if you learn information or skill in a wrong manner, how it would affect your life! Hence, just talking is not psychotherapy. These are highly structured techniques with precise goals and particular methods of administration.

During these techniques, a therapist has to follow the scientific principles without instilling his/her own values and judgment on the patient. Thus, these techniques are more than convincing to the patient. (Never say that I am fit for psychiatry because I can convince people!)

Another issue is that patient selection is very important when you are using these techniques since patient's willingness to learn these techniques is of paramount importance. Thus, psychotherapy and behavioural modification cannot be done against the patient's desire.

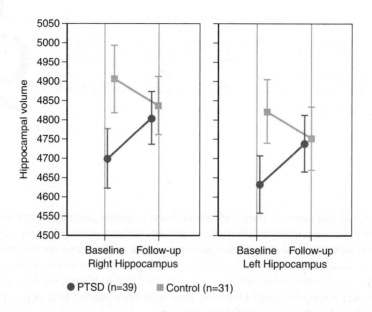

FIGURE 9.1.1

Structural changes in the brain after CBT. An increase in the both right and left hippocampal volume can be appreciated at follow up among PTSD patients.

(Source: *Levy-Gigi E. et al. (2013). Association Among Clinical Response, Hippocampal Volume, and FKBP5 Gene Expression in Individuals With Posttraumatic Stress Disorder Receiving Cognitive Behavioral Therapy.* Biological Psychiatry, *74:793–800)*

For many of these techniques, the patient has to be patient as these techniques take a long time to be learned and to be practiced (ie, to show some effect); thus, the patient must have a high frustration tolerance. Moreover, during cognitive behaviour therapy (CBT), the dysfunctional beliefs and cognitions may be revealed, which may be unacceptable to the patient. This further necessitates the need for having a high frustration tolerance.

Patients must have a 'psychological mindedness', ie, they should be able to understand their dysfunctional beliefs and their consequences while using these techniques. They must also be able to understand the outcome, if they substitute their dysfunctional belief or the behaviour with a useful one.

Besides having insight into his/her problems, the client must have the energy to practice the same outside the therapeutic sessions; hence, these are not good during acute exacerbation of psychosis or in patients with severe depression or patients who are not motivated.

A detailed description of their procedure is out of the scope of this book. Thus, we will focus on the basic principles and their uses.

COGNITIVE BEHAVIOUR THERAPY

As the name suggests, this therapy is aimed at identifying the dysfunctional cognitions (thoughts) that are translated into abnormal behaviours (acts) and modifying them using appropriate technique. This can best be understood using an example—you go to your college and you see another person who

Table 9.1.1 Emotion and Behaviour with Different Perceptions of One Incidence

Thought	Emotion	Behaviour	Rationale Thought	Emotion/ Behaviour
I always knew he was bad	Frustration Anger	Ignoring him	He appears to be busy or he must be facing some trouble, I should help him	No negative emotion or sympathy
He thinks he can control me	Despair Anger	Talking bad about him to others		
He has found new friends, now I am not important for him	Frustration Anxiety Anger Helplessness	Ignoring him Stop talking to him		

happens to be your close friend. You want to talk to the person but he/she ignores you. Now you may have a variety of thoughts related to this incidence with a variety of emotions that will determine your behaviour with the person. This is depicted in Table 9.1.1.

Thus, you have seen that one incidence can bring different thoughts, some of them may be irrational and these may influence your emotions and behaviour (first, second and third columns of Table 9.1.1). However, if you have rationale thinking, this will make your emotionally stable and your behaviour socially acceptable (fourth and fifth columns of Table 9.1.1). This is a simplified explanation of CBT.

During the therapy, the patient is asked to keep a diary of these thoughts that he/she has to bring in every session and the therapist works with the patient towards developing rationale thinking. However, you do not provide the readymade solutions to the problems, since, as a therapist, your job is to make the patient self-sufficient and capable.

RELAXATION TECHNIQUES

A number of techniques are used for the relaxation. Simplest one is deep and regular breathing or practicing 'shavasana'. However, many patients find it difficult and they may be taught Jacobson's progressive muscular relaxation (JPMR). In this technique, patients are first primed about the technique by asking them to taut one of their muscles, eg, clenching the fist as strongly as they can, and then they are asked to feel the sensation. Then they are asked to relax the clenched fist and appreciate the feeling of relaxation. You may try it yourself even right now. In JPMR, patients are made to stiffen the muscles of the neck, then relax it. In a similar fashion, they are asked to taut their jaw muscles, then of the shoulders, arms, forearms, hands, thighs, legs and feet and relax them after stiffening them for few minutes. After some practice, they start appreciating the difference. Then, depending upon the response, muscle groups may be clubbed together and they are asked to relax them in response to their mental stimulus—'relax'. The principle lies on the fact that a stressed mind and a relaxed body, or other way round, cannot coexist. Thus, with practice, patients learn to relax all their muscles in response to their own mental stimulus.

EXPOSURE AND RESPONSE PREVENTION

This technique is used to treat obsessive–compulsive disorder (OCD). These patients are made to pick any stimuli from the environment that troubles them and then respond to it in a contextually appropriate manner. For example, a patient having contamination type of OCD, has to wash his hands repeatedly when he touches anything that he *feels* is dirty. In such cases, these patients are first taught relaxation technique. Then they are exposed to such objects/surfaces and asked to relax and are encouraged to avoid acting on their compulsion (to wash their hand). Initially, patients are able to tolerate it for a few minutes, but as they practice, this time may be increased to an extent that they need not act on their obsession. This is also based on the principle of learning.

GRADED EXPOSURE/SYSTEMIC DESENSITIZATION

This is used for the patients with phobia. They are first made to learn the relaxation technique and then they make a list of stimuli, which are least frightening to them to the one that is most frightening. First, the patient is exposed to least-frightening stimulus and then you encourage him/her to relax. When the patient is able to tolerate the situation well, you take the next stimulus in the hierarchy from the list and repeat the same procedure. In this way, they learn to keep themselves relaxed even during the exposure of most frightening stimulus. This is also based on the learning technique.

PSYCHOANALYTIC AND PSYCHODYNAMIC PSYCHOTHERAPY

These are based on the psychological principles of mind. Sigmund Freud, a neurologist, but a keen observer of behaviour, proposed theories that explained how people behaved and why! In the absence of functional neuroimaging techniques, based purely on observations, he proposed that the mind has three parts—id, ego and super-ego.

According to this theory, id follows the principle of pleasure, ie, we try to get what we want. Ego works on the principle of reality, ie, what is achievable and what is not. It also tells you what is yours and what does not belong to you. Finally, there is a super-ego that follows morality. Freud postulated that our behaviour displays the conflict between these three states that are taken care of through defence mechanisms. These defence mechanisms are unconscious processes and regulate our behaviour in a particular situation. He and his successors then described that defence mechanisms can be mature or immature. For example, a person who is an artist and has sexual inclination also knows that talking about sex in the society would be immoral. Now, his mind would deal with this conflict (need to express/discuss sex and social immorality) through various defence mechanisms. One of the mature defence mechanisms is sublimation. Using this mechanism he will make nude paintings, portraits and sculptures that appear as an art to the society. These defence mechanisms are unconscious, ie, person does not know why he is doing it, but will guide his behaviour.

These theories were considered purely psychological; however, as Freud himself anticipated, we now know the neurobiology of these psychoanalytic mechanisms. Thus, they are no more psychological, instead they are biological and are governed by activity in various areas of the brain.

Id has been located to the brainstem, ego to the cingulate cortex and super-ego to the dorsolateral prefrontal and parietal cortex. Similarly, now we also know the neuroscience behind defence mechanisms. If you are interested in gaining further knowledge about it, you are advised to read the articles cited in 'references' in this chapter. These therapies require multiple session spread over years.

COUNSELLING

Counselling means providing readymade solutions related to the problem in question to a person. It is in the form of exchanging ideas or advice. Many people mistake counselling for the psychotherapy. However, they both are different from the root. Counselling does not need therapeutic alliance, whereas psychotherapy does. Counselling does not lead to a permanent change in the personality, whereas psychotherapy does. Counselling focuses on the problem in hand and you are free to advise the person, whereas psychotherapy looks at the root of the problem and you do not provide readymade advice. Counselling is influenced by counsellor's values and judgment, whereas psychotherapy is free of it. For example, if you suggest a diabetic person to refrain from sweets, it is counselling; if you advise a person with stroke or coronary artery disease to increase exercise or cut down alcohol or tobacco, it is counselling. When you explain a person about the pros and cons of undergoing surgery, it is counselling. However, it does not have any role in the treatment of psychiatric disorders, as some of the people mistakenly consider!

PROBLEM-SOLVING TECHNIQUE

This is an important technique that is useful in the situations of conflicts. After encountering a problem, some of us tend to ruminate about it (worriers), whereas others try to fight with the situation (warriors). It is a technique that helps you to measure and solve a problematic situation. It has multiple steps that are shown in Fig. 9.1.2.

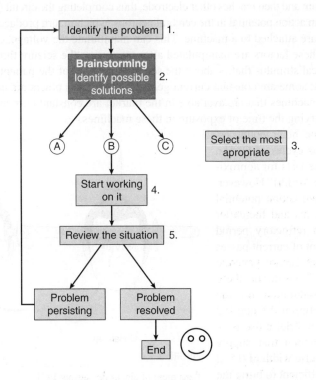

FIGURE 9.1.2

Steps of problem-solving technique.

ELECTROCONVULSIVE THERAPY

This therapy emerged after the observation that naturally occurring convulsions used to improve psychotic symptoms in patients. Cirletti and Bini were the first to develop the ECT machine. In this therapy, a brief, controlled seizure is produced by passing the electrical current through the brain, under general anaesthesia and muscle relaxants (modified ECT). EEG is recorded simultaneously to monitor the onset of seizure and its duration.

During the procedure, after anaesthetizing the patient, two electrodes are applied to the temples of the patient. A conductive gel is applied on these electrodes so as to reduce the impedance between the skin and the electrode. High impedance can result in damage to the tissue underlying the electrodes. Since, our scalp has lesser resistance as compared to the skull, most of the current bypasses the brain and reaches the other electrode. However, some of the current passes through the

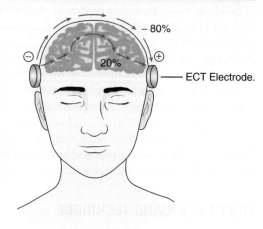

FIGURE 9.1.3

Passage of current during ECT.

skull and enters the brain and then reaches other electrode, thus completing the circuit (Figs 9.1.3 and 9.1.4). This current initiates an action potential in the cerebral neurons, which in turn produces seizure.

These electrodes are attached to a machine. This can manipulate the voltage, current and the duration of the current. These factors are manipulated after measuring the seizure threshold of the patient to produce an electrical stimulus that is above the seizure threshold of the patient. We have a number of different machines; some are constant current generators, whereas others are constant voltage generators. Most of the machines that are available in the market are constant current generators. Dose is manipulated by modifying the time of exposure in these machines.

In India and some other countries, alternative current has cycles of 60 Hz. That means, one pulse lasts for approximately 16 ms (pulse width). However, we know that neuronal action potential lasts for around 4–5 ms and thereafter neuron enters into a refractory period (Fig. 9.1.5). Thus, a lot of current passes through the brain that cannot generate any action potential. Considering these facts, optimal pulse duration for the neurons would be between 0.1 and 0.2 ms. Realizing this fact, brief pulse ECT machines were developed that supply the current with the pulse width of 0.5–2 ms. This current is sufficient to bring the

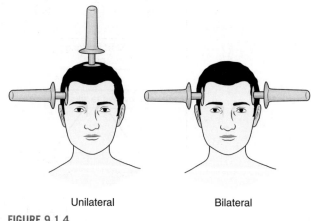

Unilateral   Bilateral

FIGURE 9.1.4

Placement of electrodes during ECT.

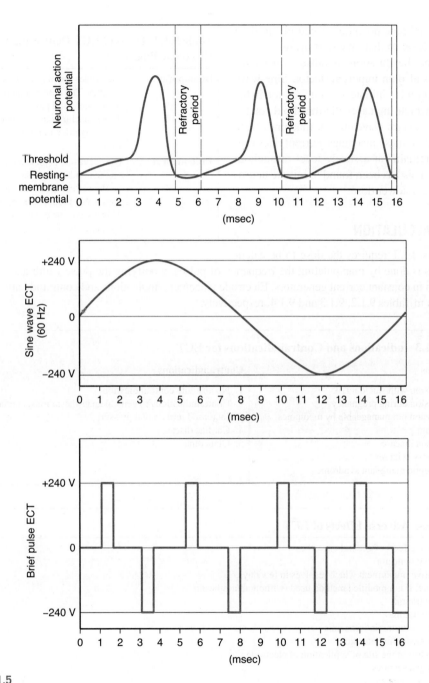

FIGURE 9.1.5

Relationship between action potential and pulse width in various ECT machines.

resting membrane potential of neurons to their threshold level so that they start firing.

Besides the duration of pulse, wave morphology is also an important factor. Sine wave has been found to initiate accommodation in the neurons, which increases the threshold for firing. Thus, square wave current machines were developed. In these machines, current rises rapidly and remains at a steady level throughout the pulse. This has been found to initiate neuronal firing at a lower dose.

DOSE CALCULATION

Like drugs, ECT requires the dose to be calculated. This is done by manipulating the frequency of pulses, modifying the pulse width and duration of pulse train in constant current generators. Electrode placement, indications and contraindications of ECT are shown in Tables 9.1.2, 9.1.3 and 9.1.4, respectively.

Table 9.1.2 Types of ECT Depending Upon Electrode Placement

Bitemporal	Electrodes are placed on both the temples. The current enters from one hemisphere and passes to the other. These machines are known to cause more cognitive impairment after ECT.
Unitemporal	One electrode is placed on the temple on the nondominant side and another on the vertex. Thus, the current bypasses the dominant hemisphere. This lessens the cognitive impairment seen after ECT.

Table 9.1.3 Indications and Contraindications for ECT

Indications	Contraindications
1. Depression with suicidal risk	1. No absolute contraindication
2. Depression during pregnancy	2. Contraindications to general anaesthesia/muscle relaxant
3. Aggression not manageable by medicines	3. Increased intracranial pressure
4. Catatonia	4. Cardiac disease
5. Parkinson disease	5. Glaucoma
6. Refractory seizures	
7. Neuroleptic malignant syndrome	

Table 9.1.4 Adverse Effects of ECT

1. Adverse effects of general anaesthesia
2. Postictal delirium
3. Cognitive impairment which resolves in few days
4. Fracture, if nonmodified method used (without anaesthesia)
5. Dental trauma
6. Muscle trauma
7. Cardiac arrhythmia/ischaemia
8. Hypertension/hypotension
9. Skin burns at the site of application of electrode
10. Prolonged seizures
11. Prolonged apnoea
12. Aspiration
13. Brainstem herniation in cases of increased intracranial pressure

MECHANISM OF ACTION OF ECT

Electroconvulsive therapy has been found to manipulate the levels of many neurotransmitters and neuropeptides in the brain including serotonin and dopamine. It also helps in neurogenesis by increasing the brain-derived neurotrophic factor (BDNF) and nerve growth factor (NGF). However, exact mechanism of the action is yet to be discovered.

REPETITIVE TRANSCRANIAL MAGNETIC STIMULATION (rTMS)

It is another method to stimulate or inhibit the neuronal activity in a given area. This is achieved by placing the coils over the scalp that produces magnetic fields. This field changes with time and this fast changing magnetic field changes (rise and fall) induced a current in the neural fields resulting in neuronal activation/inhibition. Frequencies of 1 Hz or lower are inhibitory, whereas those of 5 Hz or more are excitatory. However, r-TMS is able to change the action potential only in the cortical areas. Like mECT, dose and frequency has to be calculated. Different brain areas are targeted depending upon the neurobiology. This has been found as an effective therapy for depression (activation of left dorsolateral prefrontal cortex) and auditory hallucinations (activation of Wernicke's area) so far.

However, history of epilepsy, alcohol consumption, metallic clips inside the cranium, pacemaker and metallic prosthetic devices are contraindications to the r-TMS therapy. Adverse effects include headache and twitching of facial muscles.

SUMMARY

- Nonpharmacological therapies produce functional and structural changes in the brain.
- Adequate training is required for the administration of these therapies.
- These therapies are not psychological, rather they are biological and hence they have indications, contraindications and adverse effects.
- Nonjudicious use of these therapies may be deleterious.
- They take a long time to show their effect.
- Counselling and psychotherapy cannot be equated.
- Counselling does not have any role in the treatment of psychiatric disorders.

FURTHER READING

1. Aleman A. (2013). Use of Repetitive Transcranial Magnetic Stimulation for Treatment in Psychiatry. *Clinical Psychopharmacology and Neuroscience*, 11:53–59.
2. Berlin H. A. (2011). The Neural Basis of Dynamic Unconsciousness. *Neuropsychoanalysis*, 13:5–31.
3. Berlin H. A., and Koch C. (April 2009). Psychoanalysis Meets Neuroscience. *Scientific American* :16–19.
4. Fisher S. Z., and Student S. T. (2012). A Triple Dissociation of Neural Systems Supporting ID, EGO and SUPEREGO. *Psyence*, 335:1669.
5. Northoff G., Bermpohl F., Schoeneich F., and Boeker H. (2007). How Does Our Brain Constitute Defense Mechanisms? First-Person Neuroscience and Psychoanalysis. *Psychotherapy and Psychosomatics*, 76:141–153.

PSYCHOTROPICS: CLASSES, MECHANISM OF ACTIONS AND ADVERSE EFFECTS

10.1

Ravi Gupta

Neuropsychopharmacology deals with the study of drugs that act on the neural systems to modify the behaviour of a person. Thus, it includes the study of pathways and receptors on which these drugs act; interaction of the neural pathways with each other; and lastly, a change in behaviour that can be observed. Furthermore, it also includes the study of the pharmacodynamics, pharmacokinetics and interaction of drugs that are used for the therapeutic purpose.

However, it may be difficult to discuss everything here. Hence, we will not discuss the pharmacological properties of drugs that include names of the molecules in each class, their doses, pharmacokinetics, adverse effects and drug interactions in this section. You are advised to refer to any standard textbook on pharmacology for the same. Rather, we would like to discuss about the receptors and pathways where these drugs act. We will also discuss the neurobiological basis of their drug effect as well as their adverse effects. I will also like to discuss some general principles related to the neuropsychopharmacology.

Before we start, we would like you to appreciate that all psychotropic medicines are not the same. We have four classes of medicines that are *commonly* used in psychiatry—antipsychotics, antidepressants, anxiolytics and mood stabilizers. Besides these classes, as a psychiatrist you will also use anticholinesterase inhibitors for neurocognitive disorders, dopamine agonists and centrally acting anticholinergic for restless legs syndrome and extrapyramidal symptoms, stimulants for attention deficit hyperactivity disorder (ADHD) and many other medications, eg, opioids for opioid substitution therapy, opioid antagonists for forced withdrawal, anticraving drugs for alcohol use disorder. However, providing the neuropsychopharmacology of all these medications is impossible. So, here we will discuss only the *commonly* used drugs.

Before we proceed further, you have to understand why we are focusing on these principles rather than on pharmacology. Let us begin with an example—the antipsychotics. Though all antipsychotics appear similar with reference to pharmacodynamics, still all of them are different and this is owing to difference in their binding potential to D2 receptors. Moreover, these drugs are not selective for D2 and they act on alpha, beta, histamine and many other receptors and their subtypes, which influence their adverse effects. This is why patients have different adherence and tolerance to different drugs of same class. In addition, their pharmacokinetic properties are also different as they use different class of enzymes for metabolism—CYP2D6, 3A2 or any other subtype. It influences their drug interaction and some drugs may reach to toxic levels when given without proper information regarding its metabolism with other drugs which also influence the enzyme systems. Thus, as a psychiatrist, it is prudent that you have knowledge not only regarding receptor profile of the drug that you are prescribing (guide you to clinical effects and adverse effects) but also about the substrate of its metabolism (to prevent toxicity and to improve adherence).

PATHWAYS AND RECEPTORS

We have already discussed the neurobiology of psychiatric disorders in previous chapters. By now, you must be having an idea regarding the pathways and receptors. Here we will again discuss some basic information about these pathways and receptors.

ANTIPSYCHOTIC DRUGS

Antipsychotic drugs are also known as dopamine antagonists or neuroleptics. These drugs block D2 receptors that are responsible for their therapeutic effects as well as adverse effects. At present, we have two classes of antipsychotics—conventional antipsychotics and second-generation antipsychotics (SGA). Conventional antipsychotics are also known as first-generation antipsychotics (FGA). These drugs block only the D2 receptors. On the other hand, SGA also known as serotonin–dopamine antagonists (SDA) or newer antipsychotics, which in addition to D2 receptors, also block 5HT2A receptors that reduce the adverse effects without compromising their efficacy (Table 10.1.1).

In general, all the antipsychotics are similarly efficacious but differ in their adverse effects profile, pharmacokinetics and drug interactions, which help in choosing a drug among all of them.

We have four dopaminergic pathways in our brain—mesolimbic, mesocortical, nigrostriatal and tuburoinfundibular. Mesolimbic and mesocortical pathways originate in the ventral tegmental area and terminate into nucleus accumbens and cortex, respectively. Considering their terminal location, mesolimbic and mesocortical pathways are important for the emotion and cognition, respectively. They release dopamine that activates the postsynaptic dopamine receptors. Thus, release of dopamine in nucleus accumbens provides a feeling of pleasure, whereas it controls the cognition in prefrontal cortex. We have five types of dopamine receptors, D1–D5. D2 are present in high density in the postsynaptic neurons in nucleus accumbens and striatum. D1 receptors are mainly found in prefrontal cortex. Third pathway, the nigrostriatal pathway, starts in the substantia nigra and terminates in the striatum where released dopamine acts on D1 or D2 receptors. This pathway is responsible for motor control and any abnormality here leads to movement disorders, eg, Parkinsonism, as you all must already be knowing. Lastly, tuburoinfundibular pathway regulates the secretion of prolactin from the pituitary. Normally, dopamine inhibits its secretion. Here antagonism of D2 will increase its (prolactin's) concentration in blood. (Fig. 3.2.2)

When we give antipsychotics, they block all the D2 receptors, irrespective of their location. Thus, although dopamine is available in the synaptic cleft, it cannot act on the postsynaptic neuron. (Fig. 10.1.1)

Table 10.1.1 Antipsychotic Drugs	
Conventional Antipsychotics	**Newer Antipsychotics**
Also known as: 1. First-generation antipsychotics 2. Dopamine antagonists 3. Neuroleptics	Also known as: 1. Second-generation antipsychotics 2. Serotonin dopamine antagonists
Examples: Haloperidol, trifluperazine, pimozide, chloropromazine, fluphenthixol	Examples: Risperidone, paliperidone, qutiapine, clozapine, ziprasidone, aripiprazole, amusulpiride

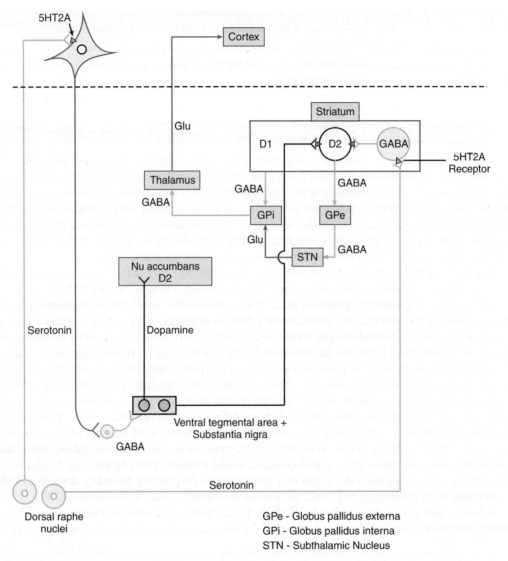

FIGURE 10.1.1

Mechanism of action of antipsychotics.

In nucleus accumbens and amygdala (mesolimbic pathway), this action leads to the clinical effects in the form of resolution of delusions, hallucinations and aggression. However, D2 blocking in other areas of the brain causes adverse effects seen with these drugs. Blocking of D2 receptors in the striatum leads to a functional reduction in the availability of dopamine, which appears as drug-induced extrapyramidal syndrome. Similarly, blocking of prefrontal cortical D2 receptors manifests as negative symptoms and cognitive impairment seen with these drugs. Lastly, blockade of D2 receptors in the pituitary causes hyperprolactinaemia (dopamine normally inhibits its secretion) that clinically

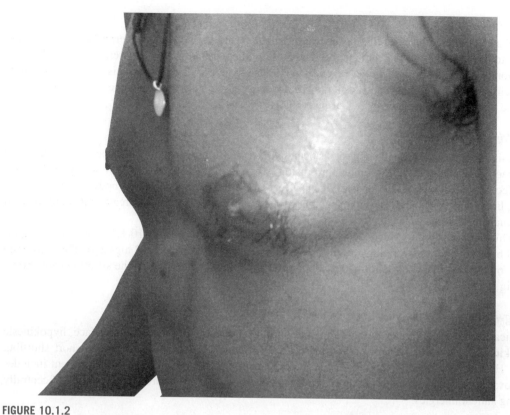

FIGURE 10.1.2

Antipsychotics-induced gynaecomastia.

(Source: Himalayan Hospital, Dehradun)

appears as galactorrhoea, decreased libido and menstrual irregularities among females. It may also induce gynacomastia among males (Fig. 10.1.2).

SDA also antagonize 5HT2A receptors (Fig. 10.1.1). Normally, serotonergic neurons from raphe nuclei send their projections to the cortex and striatum. These projections act on the 5HT2A receptors and activate the cortical glutamate neurons that project to inhibitory GABA neurons in the brainstem. These neurons inhibit dopaminergic neurons, thus causing dopamine deficiency and produce negative symptoms of schizophrenia. Through the same mechanism, serotonin reduces dopamine in the striatum, resulting into Parkinsonism. Blockade of 5HT2A through SDA reverses these actions; thus, SDA have lower propensity to induce drug-induced Parkinsonism and negative symptoms. This is also the reason why SDA are more effective in treating negative symptoms of schizophrenia.

ADVERSE EFFECTS SEEN WITH ANTIPSYCHOTICS

Like any other drugs, antipsychotic medications also have some adverse effects. Here we will focus on the neurobiological underpinnings of common adverse effects.

Hyperprolactinaemia

Blockade of dopamine receptors in tuberoinfundibular pathway leads to hyperprolactinaemia. Contrary to the striatum and prefrontal cortex, tuberoinfundibular pathway is apparently not regulated by serotonin; hence, all antipsychotics (even SDA) induce hyperprolactinaemia. This can be managed by reducing the dose of antipsychotic as it may be dose related. In other cases, change of the antipsychotic to one that has lesser propensity (eg, aripiprazole) may be effective.

Dystonia

Drug-induced dystonia usually appears as oculogyric crisis (turning of eyeballs towards one side, when it affects extraocular muscles), tongue protrusion (when it affects tongue muscles) or wry neck (when it affects sternocleidomastoid muscle). It can affect any voluntary muscle of the body including that of face, limbs and axial muscles. Laryngeal dystonia, though rare, but is a life threatening condition as it obstructs the airway.

This happens due to blockade of D2 receptors in the striatum (Fig. 10.1.1). This can be managed by giving centrally acting anticholinergic, eg, trihexyphenidyl (2–12 mg/day). This approach rests on the fact that acetylcholine and dopamine have opposite actions in the striatum (not shown in Fig. 10.1.1).

Drug-induced parkinsonism

Clinical features are similar to the idiopathic Parkinson disease and include mask face, hypokinesia or akinesia, resting tremors of approximately 2 Hz frequency, stooped posture and short shuffling gait. However, unlike idiopathic or senile Parkinsonism, symptoms are bilateral. Treatment includes removal of offending agent, if possible, and if the condition does not improve, prescription of centrally acting anticholinergics.

Akathisia

It appears as inner motor restlessness and patients feel unable to sit at one place calmly. They may keep on tapping their feet, rock their body or pace here and there without any reason. Beta-blockers (propranolol 10–60 mg/day), benzodiazepines (lorazepam 2–6 mg/day) and centrally acting anticholinergic improve the situation.

Tadrive dyskinesia

After prolonged therapy with antipsychotics (usually months to years), some patients (who are genetically predisposed) develop dyskinesia which are often limited to the face, but may be seen in other parts of the body. Common clinical presentations are chewing movements, lip smacking, repeated tongue protrusion and frowning. These are thought to be caused by super-sensitivity of the D2 receptors in the striatum. Thus, even if a small amount of dopamine is available, it induces these movements. Treatment includes prescription of high-potency antipsychotic (eg, haloperidol 5 mg/day) with gradual reduction of dose, if possible.

Neuroleptic malignant syndrome

It is a psychiatric emergency and can be lethal. Clinically, it presents as cataonia/rigidity, high fever, and fluctuating blood pressure. There may be signs of sympathetic overactivity. Often there is evidence of muscle damage and thus, serum creatinine phosphokinase (CPK) is high. Total leukocyte count may also be high. In extreme cases, muscle damage may lead to myoglobinaemia that can precipitate acute renal failure. Its pathophysiology is still not known. Treatment is mainly supportive with maintaining the hydration, cold sponging and use of centrally acting anticholinergics.

Metabolic adverse effects

SDA in particular, have higher propensity to cause metabolic adverse effects. Its pathophysiology is still poorly understood. Weight gain, dyslipidaemia and hyperglycaemia are seen with these agents. Hence, patients receiving SDA should be regularly screened for these adverse effects. It is important to measure their weight, lipid profile and blood sugar level at baseline and periodically thereof. These adverse effects consequently may lead to obstructive sleep apnoea and cardiovascular and cerebrovascular accidents.

DRUG INTERACTIONS

Drug interactions can occur at the level of pharmacokinetics or they may be pharmacodynamic interaction. These drugs are metabolized by hepatic cytochromes, so any drug that inhibits the activity of these enzymes is likely to increase the blood concentration of antipsychotics and vice versa.

Similarly, besides D2 blocking, these drugs have variable affinity for histamine (H1), acetylcholine (M1) and alpha-1 receptors. Antipsychotics antagonize these receptors. Thus, they induce sedation, have anticholinergic property and can cause hypotension. Because of the variable affinity to these receptors, the extent of their action differs. Thus, drugs that induce sedation (eg, benzodiazepines and antihistaminics), those with anticholinergic property (eg, anticholinergics and tricyclic antidepressants) and antihypertensives should be prescribed with caution along with them. Similarly, dopamine agonists and antipsychotics may compete for the receptors. Hence, they should be avoided together. For more information on this issue, you may consult a standard textbook on psychopharmacology.

ANTIDEPRESSANTS

There are different classes of antidepressants—conventional (tricyclics and tetracyclics) and newer. Newer antidepressants can also be divided into multiple classes (Table 10.1.2).

Most of the antidepressants act via blockade of reuptake of neurotransmitters, eg, serotonin or norepinephrine in the presynaptic neurons Since, selective serotonin reuptake inhibitors (SSRI) and serotonin–noradrenaline reuptake inhibitors (SNRI) are most commonly used, we will focus on their mechanism of action here (Fig. 10.1.3).

Serotonin neurons originate in the raphe nuclei. Their neurons have 5HT1A autorceptors that reduce the release of the 5HT from their terminals in various areas of the brain. These neurons also have serotonin reuptake pump in the somatodendritic region (raphe nuclei) and also at their axonal end (presynaptic) in various areas of the brain. These pumps accumulate excessive serotonin from the synapse into a vesicle in the presynaptic neurons and thus control the action of serotonin on postsynaptic neurons. SSRI block this reuptake pump; thus, the concentration of serotonin increases at the somatodendritic end. This leads to downregulation of 5HT1A autorceptors and,

Table 10.1.2 Classification of antidepressants

Classical:	
1. MAO inhibitors	Moclobemide
2. Tricyclics	Imipramine
3. Tetracyclics	Nortriptyline

New:	
1. Selective serotonin reuptake inhibitors (SSRI)	Fluoxetine
2. Serotonin partial agonist and reuptake inhibitors (SPARI)	Vilazodone
3. Serotonin antagonist and reuptake inhibitors (SARI)	Trazodone
4. Serotonin–norepinephrine reuptake inhibitor (SNRI)	Duloxetine
5. Noradrenaline reuptake inhibitors (NRI)	Reboxetine
6. Noradrenaline and dopamine reuptake inhibitors (NDRI)	Bupropion
7. Noradrenaline and selective serotonin antagonist (NSSA)	Mirtazepine
8. Melatonin agonist and selective serotonin antagonist	Agomelatine

in turn, serotonin release increases at the axonal end. It leads to the activation of intracellular cascades in the postsynaptic neurons that ultimately increase the brain-derived neurotrophic factor (BDNF) and vascular endothelial growth factor (VEGF). These factors help in neurogenesis in the hippocampal area. Increase in neurons in the hippocampus, in turn, regulate the activity of other areas of the brain, namely, dorsolateral prefrontal cortex (dlPFCx), ventromedial prefrontal cortex (vmPFCx), nucleus accumbens (NAcc), amygdala and paraventricular nucleus of hypothalamus, thus reversing the symptoms of depression (Fig. 10.1.4).

Noradrenaline reuptake inhibitors also act through the same mechanism, except the fact that autorceptors are alpha-2.

This downregulation of receptors and intranuclear changes that occur in response to these drugs, take a long time to occur. This is the reason behind the fact that these drugs do not have an immediate effect. All antidepressants are equally efficacious. The choice of drug depends upon the target symptom (whether it belongs to the dopaminergic, serotonergic or noradrenergic system), adverse effect profile and dosing schedule.

ADVERSE EFFECTS OF ANTIDEPRESSANTS

However, it must be understood that in addition to these receptors, these drugs also act on other receptors, eg, alpha-1, muscarinic receptors and histamine receptors that are responsible for their adverse effects. Alpha-1 blocking is responsible for the orthostatic hypotension; muscarinic antagonism for constipation, tachycardia, dry mouth and urinary retention and, lastly, histamine blockade for sedation and increased appetite. Classical antidepressants have more potent action on these receptors; thus, they have higher chances of these adverse effects. On the other hand, newer agents are less potent to these receptors, making them safer.

Affinity to all these receptors varies from molecule to molecule (even when they belong to the same class); thus, adverse effects differ between the molecules of even the same class.

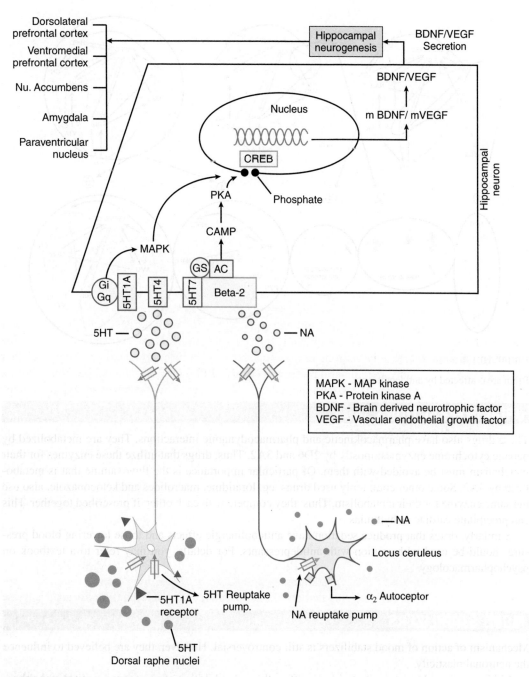

FIGURE 10.1.3

Mechanism of action of antidepressants.

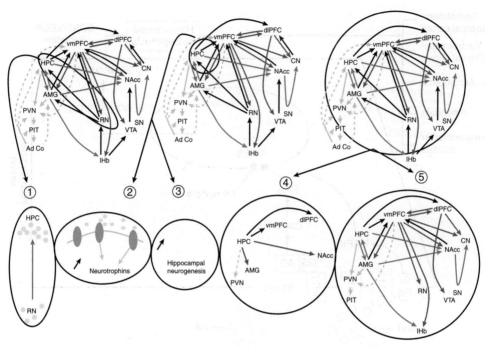

FIGURE 10.1.4

Brain areas affected by antidepressants.

DRUG INTERACTIONS

These drugs also have pharmacokinetic and pharmacodynamic interactions. They are metabolized by hepatic cytochrome enzymes; mostly by 2D6 and 3A2. Thus, drugs that utilize these enzymes for their metabolism must be avoided with them. Of particular importance is the fluvoxamine that is metabolized by 3A2. Some other commonly used drugs, eg, loratidine, macrolides and ketoconazole, also use the same enzyme for their metabolism. Thus, they compete with each other, if prescribed together. This can precipitate cardiac arrhythmias.

Similarly, drugs that produce sedation have anticholinergic effects and those lowering blood pressure should be used with caution with antidepressants. For details, you may refer to a textbook on psychopharmacology.

MOOD STABILIZERS

Mechanism of action of mood stabilizers is still controversial. However, they are believed to influence the neuronal plasticity.

Lithium is thought to exert its antimanic effect through inhibition of an enzyme inositol monophosphate and through regulation of expression of genes that influence neuronal plasticity, eg, glycogen synthase kinase-3 (GSK-3).

Valproate and carbamazepine are believed to act through inhibition of voltage-sensitive sodium channels that reduces the sodium influx in the neuron, which, in turn, reduces the glutaminergic neurotransmission.

For their adverse effect profile and drug interactions, kindly refer to a standard textbook on psychopharmacology.

ANXIOLYTICS

Benzodiazepines are most commonly used drugs for anxiolysis. These drugs bind to the benzodiazepine binding site on GABA$_A$ receptors. This site is different from the site to which GABA binds to and thus they are known as allosteric modulators (since they modulate the activity of GABA$_A$ receptors) (Fig. 10.1.5). They exert their action through positive allosteric modulation of GABA$_A$ receptors in amygdala and corticostriato-cortical loops.

SSRI exert their anxiolytic actions through 5HT1A receptors. However, their exact mechanism is yet to be elucidated. Buspirone is the partial agonist of 5HT1A and it exerts its anxiolytic action through somatodendritic and postsynaptic 5HT1A receptors (Fig. 10.1.6).

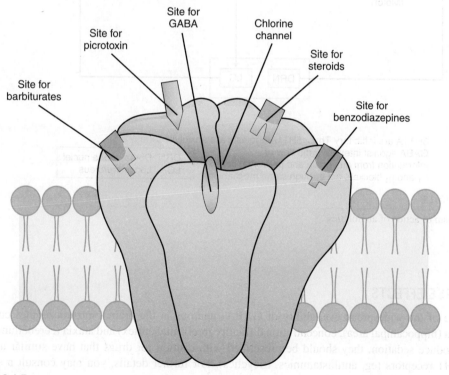

FIGURE 10.1.5

Anatomy and binding sites on the GABA$_A$ receptor.

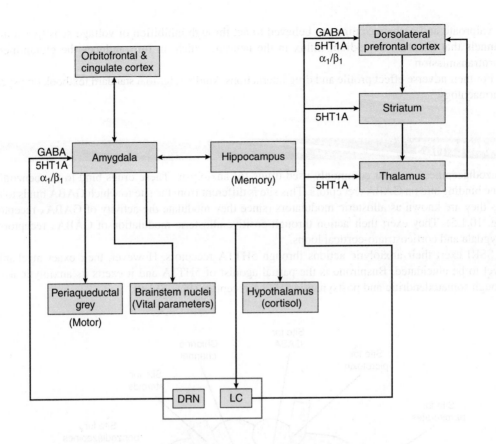

5HT1A are inhibitory. Thus, 5HT1A agouists are anxiolytics.
GABA agonist interfere c̄ the flow of
information from amygdala and prefrontal cortex.
α_1 and β_1 blockers act through same mechanism.

DRN- Dorsal raphe nuclei
LC- Locus creruleus

FIGURE 10.1.6

Mechanism of action of anxiolytics.

ADVERSE EFFECTS

Because of the widespread availability of $GABA_A$ neurons in the brain, benzodiazepines can cause amnesia (hippocampal area), concentration difficulty (prefrontal cortex) and ataxia (cerebellum). Since they produce sedation, they should be prescribed with caution for drugs that have similar action or block H1 receptors (eg, antihistaminics, tricyclics). For further details, you may consult a standard textbook on psychopharmacology.

SUMMARY

- Psychotropic drugs act to manipulate neurotransmitter system.
- They are the mainstay of the psychiatric treatment.
- They have pharmacodynamic and pharmacokinetic differences.
- They have similar efficacy but differ in adverse effect profile.
- A drug is chosen on the basis of target symptoms, adverse effect profile and dosing schedule.

FURTHER READING

1. American Psychiatric Association. (2013). "Diagnostic and Statistical Manual of Mental Disorders." 5th edit, Author, Washington, DC.
2. Stahl S. (2013). "Stahl's Essential Psychopharmacology. Neuroscientific Basis and Practical Applications." 4th edit, Cambridge University Press, Delhi.
3. Willner P., Scheel-Krüger J., and Belzung C. (2013). The Neurobiology of Depression and Antidepressant Action. *Neuroscience and Biobehavioral Reviews*. http://dx.doi.org/10.1016/j.neubiorev.2012.12.007

INTERFACE BETWEEN PSYCHIATRY AND OTHER BRANCHES OF MEDICAL SCIENCE

11.1

Ravi Gupta

Consultation liaison psychiatry (CLP) deals with the psychiatric disorders that are seen comorbid with the other medical disorders or the psychiatric disorders that present as other medical disorders, eg, fibromyalgia, chronic fatigue syndrome and irritable bowel syndrome (IBS). Sometimes, psychiatric symptoms may emerge as a result of other medical disorders or their treatment and this is also a part of CLP.

As a medical doctor, you must have the basic knowledge regarding these disorders. Like other subspecialties in psychiatry, this discipline also has its own principles that may not be contained in few pages. However, we will try to discuss all aspects of CLP without going into much detail (detailed pathophysiology, diagnostic methods and management), which is out of the scope of this book.

PSYCHIATRIC AND OTHER MEDICAL DISORDERS SEEN TOGETHER

This is a common condition and as a CL psychiatrist you may be called to examine a patient attended in medical or surgical unit for the presence of psychiatric disorder and provide appropriate therapy. It must be noted here that *psychiatric disorders are not the diagnosis of exclusion.* Thus, they should not be diagnosed just because the primary consultant is not able to diagnose any illness. This also means that these disorders may be comorbid with other medical disorders. Thus, as a CL psychiatrist, you must have the basic knowledge of the medical disorders in addition to the advanced knowledge of psychiatric disorders. This will help you in diagnosis of psychiatric disorder. For example, you have been requested by a cardiologist to provide your expert opinion regarding depression in a patient with congestive heart failure (CHF). If you have the basic knowledge regarding CHF, you will not mistake the loss of interest, fatigue, poor appetite and poor quality sleep for the symptoms of depression. These symptoms could be ascribed to inability to get engaged in work because of heart failure, gastroparesis and Cheyne–Stokes breathing seen in these patients, respectively. Moreover, adequate knowledge regarding psychiatry will tell you that the mood is not sad rather it is lethargic.

In some of the situations, you may make diagnosis of an independent psychiatric disorder and then you may decide to treat a psychiatric illness. However, you must know the adverse effects of psychotropic medications and their interaction with other medication that the patient is already receiving. For example, you may not want to prescribe imipramine to a patient with arrhythmia, benign prostatic hypertrophy or glaucoma. You may also like to avoid clozapine in a patient with psychosis associated with epilepsy who is already on valproate or carbamazepine since all these drugs are haematotoxic, and in high doses clozapine can be epileptogenic. Similarly, if you know about the interaction, you would like to avoid the fluvoxamine in patients already taking macrolides so as to avoid cardiac arrhythmias.

Moreover, adequate treatment of psychiatric disorders is also important because they may alter the course of medical disorders by influencing the adherence to treatment. For example, a depressed patient will not show adequate efforts for physiotherapy after a stroke or fracture.

Sometimes, physiological effects of the psychiatric disorders may alter the course of medical disorders and this necessitates the psychiatric intervention. For example, depression and obstructive sleep apnoea are known to induce cardiac arrhythmias in patients with myocardial infarction. Similarly, alcohol withdrawal may provoke seizures in patients with epilepsy.

PSYCHIATRIC DISORDERS PRESENTING AS MEDICAL DISORDERS

It is not uncommon for the psychiatric disorders to present as medical disorders because body–brain–mind works as one unit. Bradykinesia of depression may be mistaken for Parkinson disease; Somatic symptoms disorder-persistent pain type may be mistaken for rheumatological disorder or any other illness, eg, angina, nephrolithiasis and ureteric stone, depending upon which part of the body does it involve. Similarly, IBS may be mistaken for inflammatory bowel disease. This situation also calls for optimal knowledge regarding medical as well as psychiatric disorders while you are dealing with patients.

MEDICAL DISORDERS OR THEIR TREATMENT LEADING TO PSYCHIATRIC SYMPTOMS

Sometimes, medical disorders or their treatment may lead to development of psychiatric symptoms by inducing the neurobiological changes in the brain. This is most commonly seen with chronic infections, eg, infectious hepatitis, tuberculosis, AIDS and intracranial space occupying lesions. Chronic infections and chronic inflammatory conditions, eg, rheumatoid arthritis and systemic lupus erythematosis, are associated with a persistent inflammation in the body where proinflammtory cytokines, eg, IL-6 and IL-1β, remain high. These inflammatory cytokines reach the brain via blood and act on various centres to influence appetite, sleep, pain and fatigue. These conditions may be mistaken for depression; however, if they persist for a sufficiently long period, they may actually alter neurotransmission and produce psychiatric disorders. Similarly, intracranial space-occupying lesions (may be neoplastic, inflammatory or infectious) may interfere with normal neurotransmission and lead to the origin of psychiatric symptoms. In such cases, it is extremely important for you to have adequate knowledge of the other medical disorders so that you can rule them out before making the diagnosis of psychiatric disorder.

PSYCHIATRIC DISORDERS LEADING TO MEDICAL COMPLICATIONS

Sometimes, psychiatric disorders may lead to medical complications by altering the behaviour of the person. For example, tobacco use may lead to submucosal fibrosis and oral cancer; alcohol may lead to the hepatitis or hepatic encephalopathy; conditions associated with poor food intake, eg, major depressive disorder or schizophrenia or eating disorder, may require parenteral supplementation.

Having this much knowledge, we will now discuss common conditions that you will encounter in different departments.

GASTROENTEROLOGY

There is a close relationship between the gastrointestinal (GI) symptoms and psychiatric disorders. Almost all psychiatric disorders have GI manifestations owing to the existence of the gut–brain axis (Fig. 11.1.1).

This concept shows that gut interacts with the brain via the afferent system from the GI tract. This afferent system conveys the information related to pain and other sensations to the central nervous system, where they evoke sensory, emotional and cognitive aspects of the sensory stimulus. At the same time, efferent arm conveys the information to the GI tract and modulates activity of enteric nervous system. This model also shows that changes in the brain functioning are associated with changes in motility, secretion and blood flow of the GI tract. This is the reason behind the GI symptoms seen in psychiatric disorders.

One of the common disorders is irritable bowel syndrome (IBS). These patients present with recurrent and alternate episodes of diarrhoea and constipation. They complain of the pain in abdomen just after having food along with an urge to pass stool. They also report a change in the consistency of stool, and it is mostly liquid in diarrhoeal type, whereas it is hard in constipation type. IBS may occur due to a localized infection in the GI epithelium, sensitization of pain pathways, immunological activation in the GI epithelium and change in permeability of the intestinal epithelium. In addition to the peripheral changes, increased sensitivity towards pain, increased responsiveness to stress, neuro-inflammation in the spinal cord, enhanced neural responses to distention and structural changes in the brain have been implicated in the causation of this disorder. This is a chronic and persistent condition. This should be differentiated from inflammatory bowel disease.

Besides IBS, stress-related vagal activity has been reported to induce gastric erosions and peptic ulcers. Patients with infectious hepatitis commonly present with fatigue that may be mistaken for depression. Moreover, interferon used in the treatment of hepatitis B and hepatitis C infections may induce a variety of psychiatric symptoms, commonly anxiety and depression.

CARDIOLOGY

There is ample evidence that depression, by inducing the inflammatory mechanisms in the body, increases the risk of coronary artery disease. Depressed patients also show propensity to thrombus formation after exposure to thrombogenic stimulus, which can precipitate angina or myocardial ischaemia. Moreover, cardiac ischaemia is associated with an increment in the inflammatory activities that may induce depression in susceptible individuals. Thus, cardiac ischaemia and depression run a vicious cycle in a feed-forward manner. Depression is associated with an imbalance between sympathetic and parasympathetic systems, which may evoke arrhythmias. (Fig. 11.1.2)

Nicotine-use disorder and alcohol-use disorder are quite frequent among patients with myocardial ischaemia and they need to be addressed for the comprehensive management of myocardial ischaemia. Sleep disorders, particularly obstructive sleep apnoea, increase the risk for cardiac illness and you may be called to provide an opinion regarding that as well.

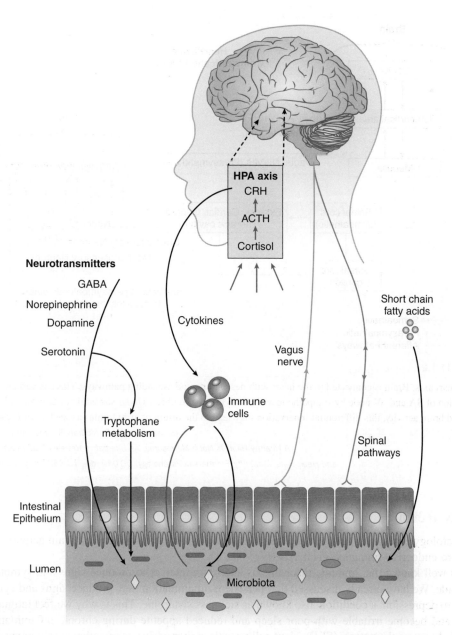

FIGURE 11.1.1

Brain–gut axis.

(Source: *Timothy G. D., Roman M. S., Catherine S., John F. C. (2015). Collective Unconscious: How Gut Microbes Shape Human Behavior.* Journal of Psychiatric Research, *63:1–9*)

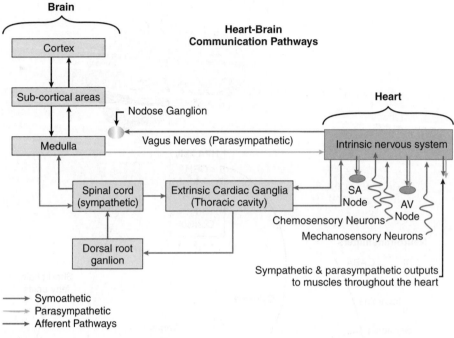

FIGURE 11.1.2

Brain–heart axis. Brain is connected to the heart with descending and ascending pathways. There is variable innervation of SA and AV node by sympathetic and parasympathetic fibres. Under stressful conditions, which lead to altered brain activity, this differential innervation may lead to the origin of arrhythmias as well as vasospasm.

(Source: Shaffer F., McCraty R., and Zerr C. L. (2014).
A Healthy Heart Is Not a Metronome: An Integrative Review of the Heart's Anatomy
and Heart Rate Variability. Frontiers in Psychology, 5:1040. doi: 10.3389/fpsyg.2014.01040)

RHEUMATOLOGY

Rheumatology deals with autoimmune diseases whose course is influenced by brain activity through the neuro-endocrino-immunological axis (Fig. 11.1.3).

It is well known that immune mechanisms and brain interact to produce signs and symptoms on either side. We have already discussed that persistent inflammation may produce signs and symptoms similar to depression, a condition also known as sickness syndrome. This is why we feel fatigued, lose energy and become irritable with poor sleep and reduced appetite during chronic inflammation, eg, systemic lupus erythematosis (SLE), giant cell arteritis, polymyositis or any other autoimmune disease. Moreover, drugs that are used to treat autoimmune disorders, eg, corticosteroids, may produce psychosis or mood disorder–like symptoms. Also, psychotropic drugs, eg, mood stabilizers and antipsychotics may cause drug-induced lupus.

Another condition for which rheumatology clinic may call the CL psychiatrist is fibromyalgia. This illness presents with pain in upper and lower halves of the body; pain on right and left sides of the body.

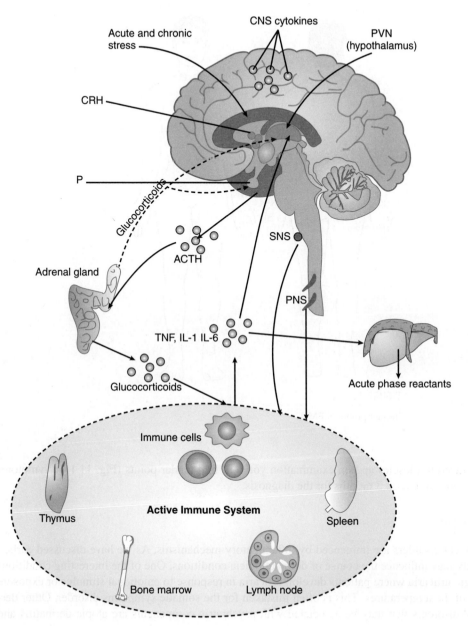

FIGURE 11.1.3

Psycho-neuro-immunological axis.

(Source: Jara L., Navarro C., Medina G., Vera-Lastra O., and Blanco F. (2006). Immune-Neuroendocrine
Interactions and Auto-immune Diseases. Clinical and Developmental Immunology, 13: 109–123)

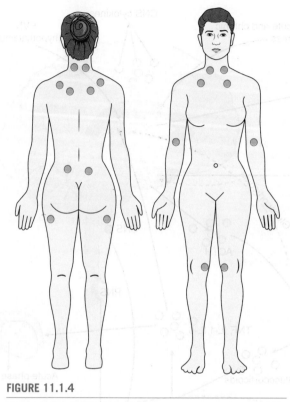

FIGURE 11.1.4

Tender points in FM 1.

Pain is localized to muscles and on examination you will find tender points (Fig. 11.1.4) Symptoms must be present for at least 3 months for the diagnosis.

DERMATOLOGY

Dermatological disorders are influenced by inflammatory mechanisms. As we have discussed earlier, brain activity may influence the course of dermatological conditions. One of the interesting conditions is cholinergic urticaria where patients develop urticaria in response to emotional stimulus or exposure to extreme of the temperatures. This is often mistaken for the somatic symptoms disorder. Other dermatological disorders that may be associated with psychiatric components are atopic dermatitis and psychogenic excoriation.

INTENSIVE CARE UNIT

As a CL psychiatrist, you may be requested to take care of the cases of altered sensorium. They are usually suffering from delirium. Sometimes, if the patient is elderly, he might be having a delirium that is superimposed upon neurocognitive disorder (dementia). Both these conditions have been discussed in detail in Chapter 5.1.

CONCLUSION

CLP is a branch where you must have the knowledge regarding both medical and psychiatric disorders. Both disorders may coexist and may influence each other. You need to be vigilant when you are dealing with this population.

SUMMARY

- Body–brain–mind acts as a unitary system and their functioning cannot be separated.
- Because of this interplay, medical and psychiatric disorders may be more frequently seen together than by chance.
- CL psychiatrist must possess adequate knowledge of the psychiatric disorders along with at least the basic knowledge of the other medical disorders.
- Adequate knowledge of psyhcopharmacology and drug interactions is the prime requirement for CL psychiatrist.

FURTHER READING

1. Jara L., Navarro C., Medina G., Vera-Lastra O., and Blanco F. (2006). Immune-Neuroendocrine Interactions and Auto-immune Diseases. *Clinical and Developmental Immunology*, 13:109–123.
2. Levenson J. L. (2005). "Textbook of Psychosomatic Medicine." American Psychiatric Publishing, Inc., Washington, DC.
3. Mayer E. A., and Tillisch K. (2011). The Brain-Gut Axis in Abdominal Pain Syndromes. *Annual Review of Medicine*, 62:381–396.
4. Shaffer F., McCraty R., and Zerr C. L. (2014). A Healthy Heart is Not a Metronome: An Integrative Review of the Heart's Anatomy and Heart Rate Variability. *Frontiers in Psychology*, 5:1040.

OLD AGE PSYCHIATRY: GENERAL PRINCIPLES

12.1

Ravi Gupta

Geriatric psychiatry deals with elderly patients. Like child psychiatry, where some of the disorders are age specific and different from general adult psychiatry, some of the disorders are seen in elderly patients that are not seen during adulthood, eg, neurocognitive disorders. Besides having some specific disorders, they physiologically differ from adult patients in a number of ways, which make them a special population. Since the clinical presentation of common psychiatric disorders encountered in this population has already been described in Section 3 on 'General Adult Psychiatry' and Section 5 on 'Neuropsychiatry', here we will focus upon some salient features that make this population different from the general adult psychiatry practice.

GENERAL PRINCIPLES

1. Neurodegenerative disorders appear with age; hence, these patients have higher chances of having neurocognitive disorders. Neurocognitive disorders and other neurodegenerative disorders must be excluded before making the diagnosis of psychiatric disorders in this population.
2. It must be remembered that the presence of neurocognitive deficits may alter the behavioural presentation of the psychiatric illnesses. Utmost care must be taken to differentiate between behavioural symptoms associated with neurodegenerative disorders and an independent psychiatric illness.
3. These patients have low neuronal reserve and hence they are at a high risk of developing delirium. This should be excluded before making the diagnosis of other psychiatric disorders.
4. These patients often suffer from other medical disorders, course of which may be influenced by psychotropic drugs. Thus, you should be extremely careful while prescribing medications to these patients.
5. These patients are often using other medications, thus you must have adequate knowledge of drug interaction before prescribing them any psychotropic agent.
6. These patients are at a high risk for adverse effects of psychotropic drugs even in the doses that are considered subtherapeutic for adults.
7. Weaker pharmacokinetic mechanisms in elderly necessitate lowering of the doses of psychotropic drugs.

8. One must have a good knowledge of medical and neurological disorders, in addition to psychiatric disorders while dealing with this population. In real world, it transforms into a multidisciplinary practice.

9. Sleep disorders, especially insomnia, is a common complaint reported by the elderly population. Always remember that total sleep time reduces with age and there are some reports that suggest advancement of circadian rhythm. Thus, you should be extremely careful while diagnosing insomnia in this population.

Although it is impossible to include every aspect of geriatric psychiatry here owing to limited scope of this book, these principles will help you in dealing with the geriatric population.

8. One must have a good knowledge of medical and neurological disorders, in addition to psychiatric disorders, while dealing with this population. In real world, it transforms into a multidisciplinary practice.

9. Sleep disorders, especially insomnia, is a common complaint reported by the elderly population. Always remember that total sleep time reduces with age and there are some reports that suggest advancement of circadian rhythm. Thus, you should be extremely careful while diagnosing insomnia in this population.

Although it is impossible to include every aspect of geriatric psychiatry here owing to limited scope of this book, these principles will help you in dealing with the geriatric population.

Index